THE OUTWARD BOUND
WILDERNESS FIRST-AID
HANDBOOK

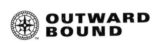

THE OUTWARD BOUND WILDERNESS FIRST-AID HANDBOOK

REVISED AND UPDATED

JEFFREY ISAAC

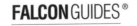

GUILFORD, CONNECTICUT
HELENA, MONTANA

AN IMPRINT OF THE GLOBE PEQUOT PRESS

To buy books in quantity for corporate use
or incentives, call **(800) 962–0973**
or e-mail **premiums@GlobePequot.com.**

FALCONGUIDES®

Copyright © 1998 by Jeffrey Isaac and Peter Goth, 2008 by Jeffrey Isaac
Previously published by The Lyons Press

Falcon and FalconGuides are registered trademarks of Morris Book Publishing, LLC.

Outward Bound is a registered trademark of Outward Bound, Inc., www.outwardbound.org

Illustrations courtesy of Wilderness Medical Associates

Library of Congress Cataloging-in-Publication Data
Isaac, Jeff.
  Outward Bound wilderness first-aid handbook / Jeffrey Isaac. — Rev. and updated.
    p. ; cm.
  Includes index.
  ISBN 978-0-7627-4513-5
  1. First aid in illness and injury—Handbooks, manuals, etc. 2. Outdoor medical emergencies—
    Handbooks, manuals, etc. I. Outward Bound, Inc. II. Title. III. Title: Wilderness first-aid handbook.
  [DNLM: 1. First Aid—Handbooks. 2. Emergencies—Handbooks. 3. Recreation—Handbooks. 4. Wounds
    and Injuries—therapy—Handbooks. WA 39 I73o 2008]
  RC88.9.O95I82 2008
  616.02′52—dc22

                                                                          2008003835

Printed in the United States of America
10 9 8 7 6 5 4 3 2 1

Contents

Acknowledgments

This book is the result of a basic idea that has enjoyed years of refinement, elaboration, and critique by hundreds of generous and thoughtful people. The original concept belongs to Dr. Peter Goth, an emergency physician with the courage, insight, and patience to promulgate a training philosophy and curriculum that truly made sense for the wilderness setting. His efforts began with the staff of the Hurricane Island Outward Bound School and later resulted in the creation and successful growth of Wilderness Medical Associates, now one of the largest wilderness medical training organizations in the world. My appreciation is extended to all of my fellow WMA and Outward Bound instructors for generously sharing their experience, comments, and encouragement. In particular, I would like to thank Dr. David Johnson, WMA's president and medical director, for his support and friendship, and for permission to use the material that serves as the foundation for much of this book. And finally to Laura, my wife and companion, I remain grateful for your patience with this itinerant medic, writer, sailor, and wilderness traveler. ✚

Introduction

The expedition is over and my students are returning to life ashore, some reluctantly, some delighted to be back. Personally, I'm looking forward to some time on my own. Teaching an Outward Bound course is an exercise in perpetual responsibility. While I accept it gladly, I surrender it equally enthusiastically when the time comes. I now have an appointment with 14 miles of upcountry white water.

The back of my pickup is packed with wet suits, gloves, piles of polypropylene, and the rest of the paraphernalia associated with spring paddling in Maine. Crowning the heap is my battered canoe. Her scars are a cumulative history of all the rocks, stumps, and other boats we've encountered over the years. In reality she is damaged equipment. But in spirit, she is a symbol of both the joys and misery of my encounters with the river.

My own bumps, bruises, and scars have healed. Fortunately, all were minor. If they weren't, I hope that I'd view them with the same degree of respect and acceptance. Risk is part of the game, and injury is one of the consequences.

This weekend thousands of paddlers will overturn their boats, climbers will fall, and hikers will become lost. The perceived risk involved in this is usually much greater than the actual danger. This is certainly true in the carefully controlled environment of an Outward Bound Program.

Nevertheless, we all understand that in many worthwhile activities there are real dangers. In Outward Bound courses we strive to balance these dangers against the joys and benefits of intimate experience with wild country and natural forces. This is the sensitive balance known as "acceptable risk."

Hazards are not sought for their own sake, but neither are they completely avoided. For backcountry travelers, a critical part of striking the balance is the ability to handle dangerous situations when they occur. This includes a logical, commonsense approach to injury and illness that takes into account the unique aspects of the wilderness setting.

In our "civilized" settings we delegate this responsibility to trained professionals. It is the business of paramedics, nurses, PAs, and doctors to recognize medical emergencies and know what to do about them. This system allows everyone else to get by with knowing very little and still keep the risk of daily living within the range of "acceptable."

But once you leave the civilized world behind, the situation changes dramatically. Techniques and equipment developed for the emergency room or ambulance are often inappropriate or impossible to use outside of the hospital. In many wilderness scenarios a team of sled dogs would be more useful than a team of surgeons.

Getting an injured person out to civilized medical care is rarely easy. Even when performed by skilled rescuers, a backcountry evacuation is difficult, expensive, and often hazardous. The popular television image of helicopters swooping to the rescue is the exception, not the rule. Even where available, safe helicopter operation is limited to a fairly narrow range of weather and terrain conditions. The "heroic" rescue is usually an arduous, sweaty, muddy scramble that disrupts the lives of dozens of people.

The object in preparing for backcountry medical problems is not to find more and better ways to scream for help, or to stuff your pack with specialty first-aid kits. It is to develop a good basic understanding of the body's structure and functions and to learn some basic techniques for preserving them in the presence of injury and illness.

It is, of course, important to recognize that there are considerable limits to your ability to affect the outcome of some medical emergencies. There are times when screaming for help is absolutely the right thing to do, and times when all the help in the world won't make any difference. The vast majority of situations, however, are well within the capabilities of every backcountry traveler to handle. It is your right and responsibility to know, at least in general terms, how your body works and how to fix it when it's broken.

Like all things remote from civilization, wilderness medicine is elemental. The most important skill is improvisation, and good improvisation requires a solid understanding of the principles behind the treatment. It's a skill like reading a river or steering a boat in a following sea. The technical information is important but it's the gut feeling for the subject that gets you through.

This book is designed to introduce the important principles, as well as to share the "gut feelings" of a lot of experienced people. It represents the collective wisdom of literally hundreds of medical practitioners, outdoor educators, sailors, and wilderness travelers. It is offered to you, not just as a reference but also as part of a lifelong process of learning. We hope that The Outward Bound Wilderness First-Aid Handbook will inspire you to further your own medical education and competence. You are, after all is said and written, your own responsibility. ✦

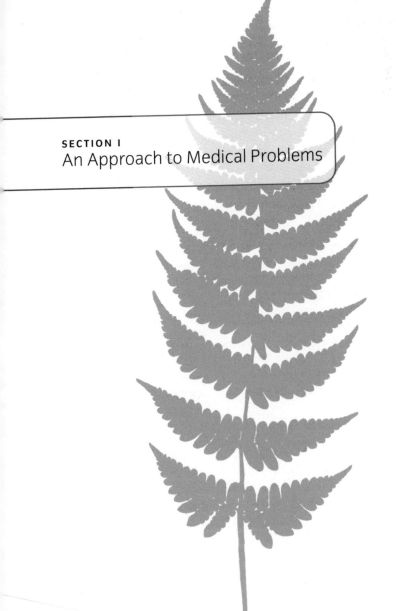

SECTION I
An Approach to Medical Problems

Chapter 1
General Principles of Wilderness Medicine

Practical preparation for medical emergencies requires truly understanding the principles behind the procedures. Once you have accomplished this, you will never "forget" what to do; you will *understand* what needs to be done. These principles are mostly common sense and basic plumbing but will turn up again and again to guide you through your study and practice of wilderness emergency care.

Oxygenation and Perfusion

The primary function of the respiratory system is to bring outside air into contact with the blood circulating through the lungs. This allows oxygen from the air to enter the red blood cells for transport to body tissues, and for waste carbon dioxide to be released from the blood and exhaled. This is called "oxygenation of the blood" and requires continuous ventilation of the lungs with fresh air.

The function of the circulatory system is to saturate all body tissues with the oxygenated blood. This is called "perfusion" and requires that the circulatory system generates enough pressure to force the blood through the miles of tiny capillaries where oxygenation of the cells and removal of metabolic waste occurs. All living tissue must be continuously perfused with oxygenated blood to function and survive.

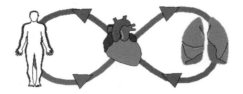

Oxygenation and Perfusion

Respiration oxygenates the blood cells.
Perfusion oxygenates the body cells.

"All living tissue must be continuously perfused with oxygenated blood to function and survive."

Adequate oxygenation of each cell in the body requires a continuous flow of fresh air to the alveoli of the lungs and a continuous flow of blood to the tissues. Anything that interferes with either of these is a serious problem. The preservation of perfusion and oxygenation is the primary purpose of emergency medical care.

Three Critical Body Systems

The organs of the circulatory, respiratory, and nervous systems perform the vital functions most essential to life. These systems are interdependent, like the legs of a three-legged stool. You can't stay upright without all three working together.

A problem with one critical system is quickly reflected in the other two. An asthma attack, for example, is a respiratory system problem that interferes with oxygenation of the blood. Under the control of the nervous system, the circulatory system will attempt to support oxygenation with an increased heart rate. If the asthma attack becomes serious, nervous system function will become impaired as oxygenation of the brain decreases.

In this case, the respiratory distress from the asthma attack is easily recognized as the original problem. In other cases involving critical system injury, it can be difficult to determine in which system the original problem lies. In any case, your ability to recognize a major problem with a critical body system is the key to recognizing a life-threatening emergency. This skill is equally helpful in recognizing when you *don't* have a medical emergency.

Three Critical Systems
Three Major Problems

Circulatory System ➡ Shock
Respiratory System ➡ Respiratory Failure
Nervous System ➡ Increased ICP

▼

"…your ability to recognize a major problem with a critical body system is the key to recognizing a life-threatening emergency."

Compensation

The nervous system regulates the function of the circulatory and respiratory systems to maintain adequate perfusion and oxygenation under a variety of conditions. Heart rate, respiratory rate, and blood vessel constriction are adjusted by the brain to compensate for effects of exercise, environment, injury, and other factors. Adequate compensation requires an intact and functioning nervous system.

The best way to watch compensation in action is by observing vital signs. The basic vital signs are pulse rate, respiratory rate and effort, level of consciousness and mental status, blood pressure, skin color and warmth, and temperature. No single vital sign is particularly valuable. But taken together, they form a pattern that can indicate good health or the development of a serious problem.

Minor changes in the pattern will occur as the healthy body adapts to the various stresses of normal life. Large or persistent changes in vital signs indicate that the body is compensating for abnormal stress, such as injury or illness. Observing the pattern and progression of vital sign changes is the best way to detect the development of a critical system problem in its early stages.

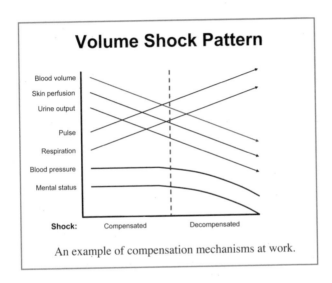

An example of compensation mechanisms at work.

The Evolutionary Onion

Nervous system tissue, including the brain, is extremely sensitive to oxygen deprivation and will often exhibit the earliest signs and symptoms of a problem with perfusion and oxygenation. The severity of the symptoms relates well to the severity of the problem. You can measure these effects by observing your patient's level of consciousness and mental status.

Picture the brain as a sort of onion with increasingly complex layers of function from inside out. The basic automatic functions such as blood vessel constriction and the control of heart and respiratory rate extend from the deeper, more primitive layers in the brain stem. Higher brain function, such as personality, judgment, and problem solving, are controlled by the outer layers of the brain. These outer layers are also the first to be affected when problems develop.

Patients remain conscious and alert but may become anxious, uncooperative, or respond in ways that don't fit the situation. Your patient may even become belligerent and confused, which can distract you from finding and fixing the problem. We sometimes call this condition "peeling the onion." Altered mental status will often be the earliest vital sign change to be seen when perfusion and oxygenation is impaired.

Swelling and Pressure

Swelling is caused by the accumulation of excess fluid in body tissues. This can occur almost instantly in the form of blood escaping from ruptured blood vessels, or slowly over hours or days as serum oozes from damaged tissue. It may be localized like the swelling of a sprained ankle, or systemic like the swelling of the whole body that occurs in allergic reactions.

Swelling that develops in a restricted space produces pressure. If the pressure is great enough, it can exceed the perfusion pressure in the circulatory system, preventing the flow of blood. This is exactly what happens if the brain swells inside the confined space of the skull, which is our major concern following a head injury. It is also responsible for the damage caused by a compartment syndrome that can develop inside the muscle compartments of the lower leg after injury. You can also create a compartment syndrome by failing to anticipate the swelling that can develop inside a splint.

Swelling in the confined space of the neck can cause an airway obstruction, preventing oxygen from getting to the lungs. Swelling lower in the respiratory system can cause lower airway constriction or pulmonary edema, which will prevent oxygenation of the blood. Any swelling that affects a major function of a critical body system is an immediate threat to life. Anticipating and controlling swelling is one of the most important aspects of long-term emergency medical care.

Ischemia to Infarction

Any body tissue deprived of its oxygen supply will die. Some tissue, like the brain, will die within a few minutes. Other tissue, like the skin, can last for hours. It seems that the more important an organ is to immediate survival, the more sensitive it is to problems with perfusion and oxygenation.

Ischemia is the term that we use for inadequate perfusion; the tissue is not receiving as much oxygen as it needs to keep working and survive. Symptoms include pain and impaired function. If the ischemia can be quickly reversed, the pain will go away and function will return.

Prolonged ischemia will inevitably lead to infarction, which is the term for tissue death. A heart attack is also called a myocardial infarction, the death of heart muscle due to prolonged ischemia. The permanent symptoms of a stroke are due to a cerebral infarction. In limb injuries, prolonged ischemia will also cause tissue infarction and permanent disability. The symptoms of ischemia are an early warning of the serious and permanent problems caused by infarction.

Ischemia to Infarction

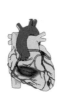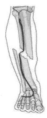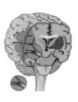

Ischemia is impaired tissue perfusion.
Infarction is tissue death due to ischemia.

"The symptoms of ischemia are an early warning of the serious and permanent problems caused by infarction."

Obstruction to Infection
The human body is full of hollow organs that store, transport, or excrete liquids of all types. These include sweat glands, intestines, bladders, and all of the associated tubing. If the drainage from these organs is obstructed by swelling, deformity, or foreign body, the buildup and pressure will cause inflammation and pain. If the obstruction lasts long enough, bacteria will begin to grow out of control in whatever substance is trapped, and infection will develop. The most common example of this principle is the teenager's worst nightmare: the average pimple. This is an infection in an obstructed sweat gland. A more serious example is appendicitis. Many serious illnesses have their origins in obstruction.

Generic to Specific
In any medical practice the process of diagnosis moves from generic to specific, with the treatment and referral following suit. But if your examining room is the salon of a small boat 200 miles offshore, getting more than a general idea of the patient's problem may not be possible. You are often left working with a generic diagnosis for the duration of field treatment and evacuation, if that becomes necessary.

The various cause of abdominal pain, for example, makes a long and complicated list. Without being in a hospital, it is nearly impossible to distinguish an ectopic pregnancy from appendicitis or any one of a dozen other surgical emergencies. Fortunately, the generic diagnosis of *serious abdominal pain* is all that's necessary to make an appropriate field treatment decision. This patient needs a hospital and your job is supportive care and urgent evacuation. In this case you don't need to waste a lot of time trying to put a specific name on something you can't treat in the field anyway.

A less serious example is a typical skin rash. You might not know specifically what it is, but you do know that it is not causing shock, respiratory distress, or impaired brain function. Your diagnosis may have to remain as generic as "rash" until you can make it go away.

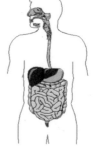

Generic to Specific

Abdominal Pain
- *Appendicitis*
- *Cholecystitis*
- *Diverticulitis*
- *Ectopic Pregnancy*
- *Etc.*

Serious or Not Serious?

"…the generic diagnosis of *serious abdominal pain* is all that's necessary to make an appropriate field treatment decision."

THE BIG NET

A corollary to the Generic to Specific Principle is the need to consider and treat all likely and possible causes of a problem until a specific diagnosis and treatment can be rendered, especially when a critical body system is involved. Altered mental status in a high-altitude climber could be caused by HAPE, hypothermia, hypoxia, intoxication, brain injury, or low blood sugar.

You must consider all of these initially, including them on the working problem list and treating accordingly. As further investigation is done and the results of treatment are observed, some of the possible causes can be ruled out and the treatment directed at those that are left. Casting the Big Net avoids the oversight caused by "puddle vision." That is, inappropriately focusing on one sign, symptom, or puddle of blood to the exclusion of all else.

IDEAL TO REAL

It is certainly helpful to have the ideal treatment in mind, but you must be able to forgive yourself for not being able to provide it. In some cases you may be able to come close. In most cases you will have to accept compromise and be willing to execute a plan that is "real" for the situation the patient is in.

The ideal treatment for a trauma patient with neck pain, for example, might involve spine stabilization with a cervical collar and vacuum mattress. But if your problem list includes being 20 meters down a crevasse in an Antarctic glacier, your patient may freeze to death before this can be accomplished. Helping the patient climb out may be the only real treatment for a situation like this.

The Risk/Benefit Ratio

There is some risk in everything we do. Medical care is no different. Every treatment or decision not to treat, and every emergency evacuation or decision to stay on expedition, involves the risk that problems will become worse because of what we've done. Against this risk we balance the potential benefits of our actions. Good decisions reflect the clear assessment that the benefit outweighs the risks to the patient and everyone else involved.

Only a major problem with a critical body system is worth a high-risk rescue. Unfortunately, there is no shortage of high-risk evacuations for low-risk medical problems. Helicopters crash and rescuers are lost in avalanches trying to evacuate patients who would have done just fine waiting a few days. In the mountains, as on the sea, it is just as important to know when you don't have a medical emergency as when you do! ✚

Chapter 2
The Patient Assessment System

Problems, by their very definition, imply a state of instability. Any problem-solving situation can be improved by the use of organizational techniques that frame the unstable problem within a stable system. In other words, trying to impose order on chaos.

In the hospital emergency department, clear priorities are established to ensure that the most life-threatening conditions are dealt with immediately by stabilizing and supporting the vital functions of the circulatory, respiratory, and nervous systems. These critical body systems include the most important and sensitive organs: the heart, lungs, brain, and spinal cord. They constitute the critical machinery most essential to life. Only after the immediate threats to the patient's life have been stabilized can a more focused assessment and treatment begin.

The same principle is followed in the backcountry setting. But because we have only our hands, eyes, and ears with which to perform the assessment, the working diagnosis and treatment tends to remain generic in nature. This makes things a whole lot easier from a medical point of view. As we've mentioned, you don't need to memorize twelve different causes of abdominal pain, you just need to know when to consider it serious.

Remember also, that in the controlled and stable environment of a hospital or clinic where most medical care is provided, the patient's medical problem is the only thing the staff needs to worry about. In the backcountry the patient's medical problem may be only a small part of a much larger picture that includes weather, terrain, the condition of the group, available assistance, and a number of other factors. Your plan needs to consider not only the medical issues but shelter, transportation, and survival as well.

In the pre-hospital and backcountry setting, an excellent tool for organized response is the Patient Assessment System (PAS). The PAS is based on information gathered in a series of surveys and organized in a standard format abbreviated "SOAP." It consists of three important steps: gathering information, organizing a response, and anticipating problems that may develop over time.

Gathering Information

The terms Scene Size-Up, Initial Assessment, and Focused History and Physical Exam describe the sequence of steps in your assessment of the scene and the patient. You may also see the terms Scene Survey, Primary Survey, and Secondary

Survey. In other publications and training programs, you may encounter different terms for similar steps in the same process. Whatever terms you choose to adopt, remember that it is the *concept* that is important.

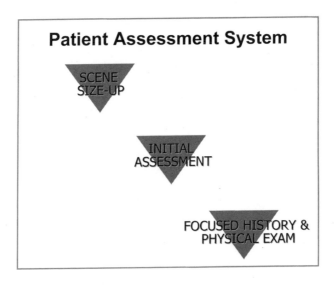

THE SCENE SIZE-UP

Rescuer and Patient Safety: Before rushing to the rescue, be sure that you are not going to create more casualties by diving into an unstable situation. You can't help anybody else if you're out of commission yourself. It can take tremendous discipline to overcome the powerful urge to come to the aid of a person in trouble. But this is exactly what you must do . . . at least for the moment. Stop, look around, and identify all of the hazards. It may be frigid water, another avalanche, or more wasps in the nest. Whatever it is, if it can harm you or your fellow rescuers, it must be stabilized before you can do anything else.

You must also consider the potential for exposure to blood and other body fluids. A number of diseases can be transmitted this way, including HIV, hepatitis, and tuberculosis. The use of gloves, eye protection, and masks is now standard in all areas of medicine where body fluid contact is possible. Protecting yourself and others from this kind of exposure is termed "universal precautions" or "body substance isolation" (BSI).

Once you are safe, or relatively so, look for any further threat to the injured person. Stabilize the scene by moving danger from the patient, or the patient from the danger. This has priority over everything else that follows. So, get him out of the water, out from under the cornice, or away from the wasps before proceeding with evaluation and treatment.

Mechanism of Injury: Another important element in the scene size-up is determining the mechanism of injury. How it happened is usually obvious, but occasionally more investigation will be necessary. For example, how far did he fall? Was it enough of a tumble to cause significant injury? Are there other factors, such as exposure to weather or pre-existing illness, that might be the cause of the patient's condition?

Number of Patients: Determine how many people are injured or at risk. Potentially serious problems are often overlooked in the rush to treat the most noisy and uncomfortable patients. This is especially true in harsh environments where all expedition members are at risk for hypothermia or dehydration.

Triage, which is the process of establishing treatment priorities, is important in multiple casualty situations where resources are limited. This is a good time to avoid "puddle vision." Look beyond that puddle of blood right in front of you and size up the whole scene before deciding where to apply what help you have to offer.

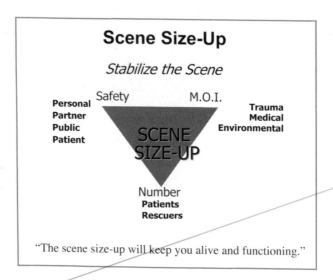

THE INITIAL ASSESSMENT

This is your initial quick-check on the status of the patient's three critical body systems. The critical functions of the circulatory, respiratory, and nervous systems are equally important to survival, and serious problems are equally life-threatening. The order in which you check and stabilize them will be determined by the situation, not by the order in which they appear on any list.

Make sure that the mouth and nose are clear to allow the passage of air, and that air is actually going in and out. Be sure that blood is circulating and not running out all over the ground. While you are doing this, ensure that the patient's spine is stable, and check the level of consciousness.

Performing an initial assessment may mean hanging upside down in a crevasse listening for breath sounds in your unconscious partner and looking inside bulky clothing for blood. On the other hand, it may be as simple as asking "how do you do?" and getting a "fine" and a smile. Whatever form it takes, it is a critical step in your organized approach to the situation because any problems encountered in the initial assessment must be immediately stabilized before worrying about anything else. You will have to fight the natural tendency to focus on the obvious injuries like deformed fractures and messy abrasions. This can keep you from finding the life-threatening problems, such as airway obstruction or severe bleeding. Remember the Big Net Principle!

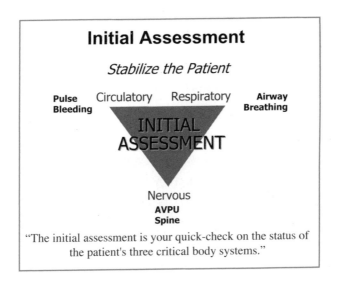

Initial Assessment

Stabilize the Patient

| Pulse
Bleeding | Circulatory | Respiratory | Airway
Breathing |

INITIAL ASSESSMENT

Nervous
AVPU
Spine

"The initial assessment is your quick-check on the status of the patient's three critical body systems."

The immediate management of life-threatening problems found in the initial assessment is referred to as Basic Life Support (BLS) and is covered in chapter 3. If the situation requires BLS, you may never be able to go any further with your patient exam. In most cases, however, you will be able to determine that no life-threatening problem exists and go on to the Focused History and Physical Exam.

FOCUSED HISTORY AND PHYSICAL EXAM

By now you have decided that neither you nor the other rescuers or the injured person is in immediate danger from the environment around you. The patient has no critical body system problems that are going to kill him right now. For the moment the scene is stable, and the patient is stable.

Focused Physical Exam: This stage is a slower and more deliberate examination of the whole patient. It is less urgent than the initial assessment, but speed and detail change with circumstances. Unless your initial assessment missed something, it is not necessary or efficient to stop and treat problems as you find them. Get the whole picture, complete your list, and then return to treat each problem in order of priority.

Although it really makes no difference in what order you do your exam, most people like to start with the head and neck, moving to the chest, abdomen, pelvis, legs, arms, and back. You are looking and feeling for abnormality such as tenderness (pain caused by touch), swelling, deformity, discoloration, or bleeding. You should be gentle, moving the patient as little as possible.

Your exam should be as comprehensive as the situation allows and requires, but common sense should prevail. It is not always necessary to directly see or feel every body part in every patient. If no symptom or mechanism of injury suggests involvement of a particular body part, exposure and examination is not important, especially in the field. What is important is that the rescuer go through a complete head-to-toe checklist, at least in his own mind.

Focused History
and Physical Exam
Complete Then Treat

Physical Exam   SAMPLE History

FOCUSED HISTORY
& PHYSICAL EXAM

Vital Signs

"Get the whole picture, complete your list, then return to
treat each problem in order of priority."

Vital Signs: While the initial assessment looks quickly for urgent problems with the circulatory, respiratory, and nervous systems, the vital signs provide more objective measurement of these same three systems over a period of time. Changes in the function of the critical body systems will be revealed by changes in vital signs, often following predictable patterns. You can think of vital signs as the "safety net" of patient assessment. They can serve to reassure you that the patient is OK, or provide an early warning of developing trouble.

By measuring the same standard signs at regular intervals, you can get a sense for improvement or decay in a patient's condition. Is your treatment working? Are things getting better or worse? Is it time to panic, or can you sit back and have another handful of gorp?

The detail with which you measure vital signs will depend on the equipment available and your level of training. How often you measure vital signs will depend on the logistical situation and your level of comfort with the patient's condition. Vital signs are listed below, with the range of normal values in parenthesis.

Pulse is a very helpful and reliable vital sign; it is easy to measure accurately and reflects almost any change in the circulatory system. Pulse rate is expressed in beats per minute and can be quickly obtained by counting the pulse for fifteen seconds and multiplying by four. Noting the rhythm (irregular or regular) can be helpful in some cases, but subjective comments like "weak," "thready," or "bounding" are rarely useful. You can find the pulse in any artery, but the radial (wrist), carotid (neck), and temporal (temple) are the most commonly used.

Respiratory rate is a direct measurement of respiratory system function but can be difficult to measure accurately if the patient is talking or crying. It is expressed in breaths per minute as well as noting the degree of effort involved in breathing.

Blood pressure, like pulse, is a direct measurement of circulatory system function. A reading of 120/80 would be normal for an adult. The first number (systolic) indicates the pressure produced by the force of each heart contraction. The second (diastolic) reflects the resting pressure of the system maintained by arterial muscle tone. For emergency use, the systolic pressure is the easiest to obtain and the most useful.

Vital Sign Pattern

P - Pulse: note rate and if regular or irregular
  (adult resting rate: 60-100/min.)
R - Respiration: note rate and effort
  (normal adult: 12-24/min, and easy.)
BP - Blood Pressure: systolic/diastolic
  (normal: 100-140, diastolic; 60-90)

"While the initial assessment looks quickly for urgent problems, the measurement of vital signs provides a more complete view of critical system function and compensation."

Systolic blood pressure is measured by inflating a blood pressure cuff around the upper arm or leg and applying enough pressure to completely stop arterial blood flow. The cuff is then slowly deflated while the examiner watches the gauge and feels for the return of the pulse in the wrist or foot. The reading on the gauge when the first beat is felt is the systolic BP. To obtain the diastolic pressure, a stethoscope is required to hear the change in sounds that occur within the artery as the cuff pressure is lowered.

Vital Sign Pattern

T - Temperature (normal core temp 37° C)
S - Skin: color, temperature, moisture
AVPU - Level of Consciousness:
- A - awake, further define mental status
- V - responds to verbal stimulus
- P - responds to pain stimulus
- U - unresponsive

"The awake patient is further described in terms of mental status using terms like oriented, disoriented, confused, combative, and so on."

Temperature as a vital sign refers to the temperature of the vital organs of the body core. This can be quite different from skin temperature, even in the normal patient. The most accurate place to easily measure core temperature is in the rectum. Oral temperatures are affected by eating, breathing, and talking and are usually about a degree lower than core temperature.

Skin color and temperature are a measurement of shell perfusion, that is, blood flow to the skin and less vital organs. It is described according to skin color, temperature, and moisture. Skin perfusion is reduced whenever vital organ perfusion is reduced. However, cool and pale skin can also be part of the normal response to cold weather.

Level of consciousness and mental status is a measure of central nervous system function, specifically the function of the brain. No special instruments are required. Consciousness is described as relating to one of four letters on the AVPU scale.

AVPU is a widely used and precise description that avoids confusing terms such as "semiconscious" and "in and out." You can fine-tune your description of a patient who is awake by describing mental status. This refers to the level of orientation and anxiety. Serious problems in the critical body systems almost always cause some change in mental status well before changes in consciousness.

People with normal mental status generally know who they are, where they are, what day it is, and the purpose for their being there. You'll have to allow some slack for time at sea, of course. We've had perfectly healthy Outward Bound students on long expeditions unable to keep track of the month, never mind the day of the week.

When measuring vital signs, it is most important to take them together at regular intervals and record the time they were taken. Remember, the value of this assessment "safety net" is in observing change over time. Even if you don't carry blood pressure cuffs, clinical thermometers, or even a watch, a valuable assessment of vital signs can still be made. Measurements become relative; for example, pulse is "fast" or "slow," temperature is "cool" or "warm." Blood pressure can be assessed as "normal" or "low" based on signs of adequate or inadequate perfusion (more on that later).

History: This is the process of gathering information about what happened and what other influences there might be on the current condition. The acronym for what to ask is abbreviated **SAMPLE:**

SAMPLE History

S – Symptoms:
- Onset and progression
- What makes it better or worse?

A – Allergies:
- To medications, food, environmental allergens
- Note type and severity of previous reactions

M – Medication:
- Prescription, over-the-counter, homeopathic
- Vitamins

P – Pertinent History:
- Previous similar symptoms or problems
- Contributing factors

L – Last Ins and Outs:
- Food, fluids: time and quantity
- Urine and bowel, normal or abnormal
- Last menstrual period

E – Events:
- Leading up to the accident or illness
- Consider mixed mechanisms

In a complicated illness or multiple trauma, performing a focused history and physical exam can take some time. Many accident scenarios are not witnessed, confused by pain and anxiety, and involve hidden injuries. In these situations your level of anxiety as a rescuer can be reduced by having a familiar structure to function within. You are also more likely to find and fix the important problems. Using the Patient Assessment System will do a lot to put your mind at ease and stabilize an uncomfortable situation.

With simple cases your PAS can be very brief. A finger laceration doesn't warrant a full body examination or a discussion of the patient's gall bladder surgery fifteen years ago. The survey of most backcountry medical problems is short and sweet.

Organizing Your Response

The system of organization and communication commonly used by the medical profession is the **SOAP** format. SOAP is the acronym for *Subjective, Objective, Assessment,* and *Plan*. It is a simple and effective management process from the gathering of information, through the identification of the problems, to the formation of a plan to deal with each problem. It is the way medical records are written and communicated. The general meaning of each heading is as follows:

Subjective: Description of the scene, the mechanism of injury, symptoms the patient is complaining about, relevant history (SAMPLE).

Objective: What you see, hear, feel, and smell during your examination of the patient. Includes vital signs.

Assessment: The "problem list" based on the subjective and objective findings.

Plan: What are you going to do about each problem now? This includes treatments, plans for monitoring the patient's condition, and plans for evacuation if necessary.

Using this system, a typical brief SOAP for an emergency department case might look like this:

S: A nine-year-old boy fell off his bicycle when he rode over a curb at slow speed. He complains of pain in his right wrist and tingling of his fingers. He has no complaints of pain anywhere else. No allergies, no medications, no past history of wrist injury, last meal noon, fell because he didn't see the curb.

O: An alert, oriented, but uncomfortable boy. The right wrist is swollen and tender to touch. There is no other obvious injury. The patient refuses to move the wrist voluntarily. The fingers are warm and pink and can be wiggled with slight pain felt at the wrist. The patient can feel the light touch of a cotton swab on the end of each finger. X-ray shows a buckle fracture of the distal radius (minor break in the end of one of the bones in the forearm).

A: Fracture right wrist.

P: Splint wrist. Follow up with an orthopedic surgeon in three days. Return to the hospital if fingers become blue or cold or the tingling becomes at all worse.

This format paints a nice picture of the situation. In just a few words, you get a sense for who the patient is and what happened, and what the practitioner is going to do about it. There is also a brief description of problems that might occur and what the response should be.

The SOAP format is perfectly adaptable to the backcountry setting, and it performs the same vital function that it does in the emergency department. It organizes your thoughts, renders order from chaos, and allows you to communicate your ideas and plans to the patient and whoever might be taking care of the patient next.

In the wilderness setting we need to expand SOAP to take into account the unique environment in which we are traveling. In addition to the injury, we must also consider problems created by weather, terrain, distance, and time. These factors are just as important to our planning as the condition of the patient. In long-term care we add a list of "anticipated problems" (A'), which could be complications of the injury itself or the result of exposure to environmental factors. By including A' in the SOAP note, we are more likely to prevent problems from developing or be ready to deal with them when they can't be avoided.

As your patient's condition, the weather, and your logistical situation changes with time, plans will need to be revised and communication updated. You will want to repeat the relevant parts of your surveys and revise your SOAP at regular intervals. This is where you watch for the anticipated problems (A') you've listed in your original SOAP note.

Patients with potential critical body system problems should be reevaluated most often, at least every ten minutes if possible. The status of injured extremities can be checked less frequently at one- to two-hour intervals. Conditions that develop slowly, such as wound infection, might be adequately monitored every six hours.

Now, with these specialized additions to SOAP in mind, let's take that previous emergency department case into the backcountry:

S: A nine-year-old boy fell onto his outstretched right arm while gathering firewood near the Speck Pond Shelter about one hour ago. He complains of pain in his right wrist and tingling in his fingers. He has no complaints of pain anywhere else. No allergies, no medications, no past history of wrist injury, last meal noon. The fall was due to slipping on wet leaves and not from a significant height. He does not feel cold or hungry. It is now sunset. The air temperature is 60 degrees. It is raining lightly.

O: At 18:30, an alert, responsive but uncomfortable boy is found sitting on a rock holding his right arm. He is warm, dry, and adequately dressed. His right wrist is slightly swollen and tender to touch, and he is unable to move it. He can wiggle his fingers and feel the light touch of the examiner's hand. His skin color is normal. There is no other obvious injury.

A: Unstable injury right wrist.

A': 1. Increased swelling, pressure, ischemia

   2. Hypothermia

P: Splint the wrist, keep the patient quiet and the arm elevated.

   1. Monitor right hand every two hours, adjust the splint if necessary.

   2. Stay in shelter tonight, walk out in daylight tomorrow.

In this example the anticipated problem of hypothermia is included because it often occurs in wet and cool weather, especially in a person who is not exercising and eating well. By listing it as an anticipated problem, we are reminded to take measures to prevent it. This is a perfect use for the anticipated problem list.

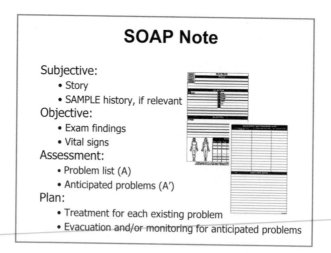

In more complicated cases where a patient may have more than one problem, the format remains the same. Under A (Assessment) we would list the problems in order of priority, and be sure that we have a plan for each one. By checking each problem for a plan and each plan for a problem, we can avoid missing anything. We can also avoid the very common practice of making plans for problems that don't exist. ✚

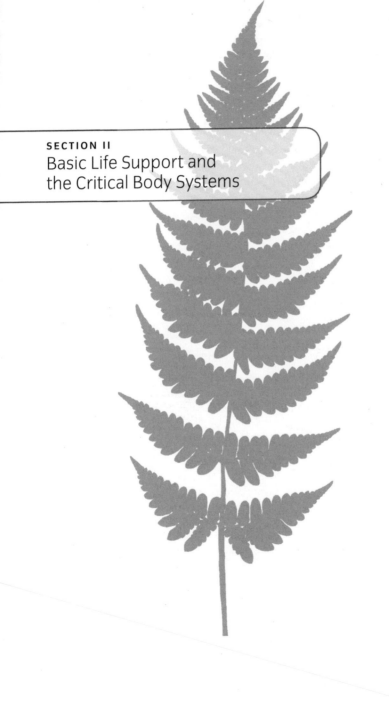

Chapter 3

Basic Life Support

Discussing serious problems first has its drawbacks. You can get the feeling that every accident is going to produce some tragic and overwhelming injury. It can make you a bit shy about taking risks, or even letting yourself get more than a mile or two from a Level I trauma center. So please keep in mind that we cover the big problems first because they're big, not because they're common.

Basic Life Support (BLS) is the immediate treatment of life-threatening critical body system problems discovered during the initial assessment. The goal is to support oxygenation and perfusion while patient assessment continues. For BLS to be effective, it must begin immediately at the scene.

In terms of saving lives, all BLS components are equally important. Although BLS is outlined in a specific sequence, field treatment requires flexibility. It is often necessary to change the order in which things are done or to manage several components at the same time.

Most of the procedures involved in basic life support are covered by the obstructed airway and cardiopulmonary resuscitation (CPR) courses taught by the American Heart Association, Red Cross, WMA, and other organizations. We strongly recommend your participation in one of these courses, although it will require some flexibility to adapt what you learn there to the wilderness environment.

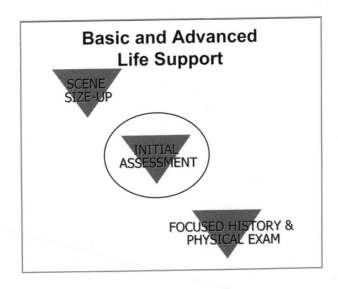

You'll remember from the chapter on the Patient Assessment System that the initial assessment is a rapid check on the function of the circulatory, respiratory, and nervous systems. The easiest way to do this is to ask the patient, "Hey, how are you?" If he gives an appropriate verbal response, such as, "Fine, will you help me get this rock off my foot?", you can be satisfied that there is no immediate life-threatening critical system problem. He is breathing, his heart is beating, and his brain is functioning. You have done your initial assessment. In cases where the patient is unable to respond or has responded abnormally, you will need to look a little more closely.

BLS for the Respiratory System

Is your patient moving enough air in and out to adequately oxygenate the blood? A person who is able to speak generally has ventilation adequate for the initial assessment. A patient who can carry on a conversation is in pretty good shape from a respiratory point of view. Even in the presence of respiratory distress, a brain that is functioning more or less normally is an indication of adequate oxygenation.

If your patient is working so hard to breathe that talking is difficult or impossible, or you are seeing significantly altered mental status or level of consciousness in the presence of respiratory distress, you are dealing with a life-threatening emergency called respiratory failure that must be treated immediately. The generic treatment for respiratory failure is abbreviated PROP and will be discussed in more detail in chapter 5.

If you are unsure about respiratory status, you might have to fall back on your own experience. You have a great deal of experience with breathing; you have been doing it ever since you were born. If you don't think your patient is breathing well enough, she isn't. This is reason enough to begin to support ventilation with mouth-to-mouth or mouth-to-mask.

Respiratory failure or arrest is treated by blowing into the lungs through the airway. This is called positive pressure ventilation (PPV). The rate of ventilation should be twelve breaths per minute, or about one every five seconds. If you don't like counting, just start the next breath as soon as the patient has finished exhaling. Blow in enough air to cause the chest to rise slightly. Each breath is done slowly over one to two seconds. Faster flow rates tend to blow air into the stomach, causing distension and vomiting.

Patients who are breathing on their own but not deeply or frequently enough can be assisted with PPV timed to blow air in with the patient's own inspirations. This is especially useful in treating inadequate respiration due to chest wall injury. Even if you can't time your ventilation exactly, a patient in trouble will quickly adjust to your efforts.

If you are unable to get air into the lungs, the problem may be upper airway obstruction. You may have already picked up some clues in your survey of the scene: dinner time, steak and potatoes, clutching her neck . . . that sort of thing. Other causes of obstruction include swelling, spasm, position, and deformity from trauma.

Clearing an airway obstruction is a progression of actions from the most simple to the most desperate. The airway is opened by gently extending the neck and lifting the chin, or pulling the jaw forward away from the throat (jaw thrust). If these positioning maneuvers do not allow for breathing or ventilation, you must try to clear the obstruction manually.

It is a perfectly natural reaction to want to look inside the mouth to figure out what's wrong. Go ahead; you may see a foreign body that can be pulled out with your fingers or a clamp. If there's nothing to see, try using the residual air in the patient's lungs to help clear the obstruction. A firm thrust to the abdomen or chest can force the air left in the patient's lungs out under pressure, blowing any obstruction out with it. The abdominal or chest thrust is done with the patient on her back. In cases where an obstructed patient is still conscious and standing, it is done from behind by grasping your own arms around the patient and squeezing. It really doesn't matter whether you are squeezing the abdomen or the chest, the effect is the same.

Another technique is a firm back blow between the shoulder blades. This method has fallen out of favor in standardized training except for use with infants. But it works on adults, too, and should be considered if abdominal thrusts are not working.

Respiratory Failure

Basic Life Support:

Position for easiest respiration.

- Clear airway, position for drainage
- Nasopharyngeal and oropharyngeal airway use, suction

Reassurance to improve respiration.

Oxygen via mask or nasal cannula.

- Titrate to response
- Heat and humidify

Positive Pressure Ventilation.

- Can be effective for hours or days
- Can be used to assist inadequate respiratory effort

If the obstruction is due to swelling of the airway, back blows and abdominal thrusts will not help. Your best treatment will be to continue PPV in an attempt to force air past the obstruction while repositioning the neck for the best air flow. Airway swelling is best treated with medications or rapid extrication to advanced medical care where a surgical airway can be established.

BLS for the Circulatory System

Cardiac arrest means the loss of effective heart contractions. In your initial assessment, you are checking for the presence or absence of a pulse. Because cardiac arrest immediately causes respiratory arrest and complete loss of consciousness, we can be confident that any patient who is at all responsive, breathing, or moving spontaneously is not in cardiac arrest.

The pulse can be very difficult to find under adverse field conditions where you may be working with cold hands in dangerous places. The pulse can be weak or absent in the extremities of a person in shock, and very slow in profound hypothermia. It is extremely important to take the time to find a pulse. The carotid and temporal pulses are the easiest to get to and always present if the heart is beating. The carotid is located on either side of the larynx (Adam's apple) in the neck. The temporal is on the side of the head just in front of the ear.

Cardiac arrest is treated temporarily with cardiopulmonary resuscitation (CPR), which is a combination of chest compressions and PPV, which allows some oxygenation and perfusion of the brain and vital organs. The technique has been learned by millions of people and has saved many lives in settings where Advanced Life Support (ALS) and hospital care are available within a few minutes.

For CPR to be effective, the patient's critical systems must still be intact. CPR will not support perfusion in cases where the cardiac arrest was caused by massive trauma or shock. CPR will not work if the arrest was caused by brain or spinal cord injury. The survivors of cardiac arrest are typically patients who have experienced ventricular fibrillation or other cardiac arrhythmia due to a heart attack and were lucky enough to have quick access to CPR, defibrillation, an ambulance, and a hospital.

In the United States and other developed nations, automatic external defibrillators (AED) are now installed in airports and bus stations and being carried in police vehicles. The idea is to initiate CPR and defibrillation within the first five minutes while the heart has some chance of responding. The AED is designed to electrically stop a fibrillating heart in hopes that it will restart in its normal rhythm.

Any reasonable chance of survival with CPR and an AED further depends on immediate treatment with drugs or electronic pacing to stabilize the heart rhythm, and medical or surgical care to correct the underlying problem. This system does save lives in urban areas. The best of such integrated medical systems have achieved cardiac arrest survival-to-discharge rates of around 20 percent.

Unfortunately, CPR and defibrillation have very limited application without access to ALS and hospital care. CPR by itself will not restore normal cardiac rhythm, and defibrillation alone will not fix the cause of the arrest. The chance of a successful resuscitation without definitive medical care is remote. As of this writing, there are no documented saves using an AED in the backcountry or offshore setting without access to follow-up care.

Most of the successes attributed to CPR probably occur in cases where the heart was not actually in arrest. It is also possible that a cardiac arrest caused by respiratory failure due to events like asphyxia or lightning strike could be reversed by prompt oxygenation of the lungs and chest compressions. These cases offer the best chance for a successful resuscitation, and a good reason to perform CPR in any setting.

Cardiac Arrest
WILDERNESS PROTOCOL

<u>Do Not BEGIN CPR:</u>
- Obviously dead from lethal injury
- Submerged under H_2O greater than 1 hour
- Trauma with no pulse

<u>Start CPR and ALS otherwise*</u>

<u>STOP CPR:</u>
- Spontaneous pulse resumes
- Authorized medical professional pronounces the patient dead
- Rescuers are exhausted or at risk
- After 30 minutes of sustained cardiac arrest

* See Thermoregulation for recommendations specific to severe hypothermia.

Even under the best of circumstances, CPR can only support oxygenation and perfusion for a very limited time. The chances of recovery after thirty minutes of sustained cardiac arrest are zero, with the possible exception of severely hypothermic patients. For this reason, WMA Wilderness Protocols call for CPR to be discontinued after thirty minutes of pulselessness.

Even with a strong pulse, adequate perfusion requires adequate circulating blood volume. Severe blood loss must be controlled as part of the BLS process. Bleeding can be external and obvious, or internal and hidden. Even profuse external bleeding can be missed when a full exam is not done. Snow and bulky clothing can absorb or obscure blood. This can be a real problem when the clothing is waterproof and the weather is too extreme to permit undressing the patient.

Bleeding from an artery is the most immediately life threatening. It will be under pressure and may spurt with the pulsing of the heart. There is no definite way to decide when bleeding is severe. If it looks like a lot of blood, it probably is.

Unfortunately, internal bleeding is not so obvious. It should always be suspected with a history of trauma and the development of shock. Severe internal bleeding is usually associated with fractures of the femur and pelvis and blunt abdominal and chest injury.

External bleeding is controlled by well-aimed direct pressure over the bleeding site. Pressure can be applied with a gloved hand if necessary, but a bandage or cloth should be used. This is not so much to absorb blood as to provide even pressure across the damaged vessels.

If bleeding continues, remove the bandage and look again for the source of blood. Re-aim your pressure. You should expect to apply pressure for fifteen or more minutes before a clot will form. Once bleeding is controlled, a pressure bandage should be applied. Beware, however, of obstructing circulation by creating an accidental tourniquet.

A tourniquet can be used when you want to completely obstruct circulation to a limb when there is no other way to stop bleeding or when there is no time to do so. This may be necessary in mass casualty disasters and unstable and dangerous scenes such as fire fighting or combat. The tourniquet can be removed and the bleeding controlled by direct pressure when a safe zone is reached or the patient's other initial assessment problems are stabilized. A tourniquet should not be left in place for more than an hour or so or the intentional ischemia will result in unintentional infarction.

Severe internal bleeding, indicated by pain and the onset of volume shock, is difficult to control without surgery and is likely to be fatal in the wilderness setting. Less severe internal bleeding may be detected by the gradual onset of compensated shock and the progression of pain. In these cases early recognition and evacuation may be lifesaving.

BLS for the Nervous System

Fracture or dislocation of the bones of the spinal column can damage the spinal cord with dramatic, devastating, and permanent results. Reducing the risk of further injury to this vital structure is considered part of BLS. The most dangerous movement for a damaged cervical spine is flexion (movement of the chin toward the chest). Moderate extension is usually safe. Hyperextension (tilting the head back) is also considered dangerous.

Nervous System Failure

<u>Basic Life Support</u>:

Spine Stabilization Unless
- No mechanism of injury
- Increases risk to patient or rescuers
    - inhibits extrication from unstable scene
    - increases evacuation hazard
    - Impairs other critical system treatment

"If no movement of the spine is required for life saving treatment, leave the patient where he is while you complete your assessment."

Any trauma that could produce spine injury is called a "positive mechanism." This is determined during your scene size-up. Examples include a fall from a cliff, being tumbled by an avalanche, or a short swim over a long waterfall. No further spine exam is necessary during the initial assessment; these are all treated as spine injuries for now.

If no movement of the spine is required for lifesaving treatment, leave the patient where he is while you complete your assessment. If you must move the spine, bring the head and neck into the neutral, eyes-forward position. Stabilize the head and neck in this position during BLS and the rest of the patient survey. Spine splints, if necessary, are applied after the PAS is finished.

The airway can usually be kept clear of obstruction with the neck held in the neutral position. If it is necessary to roll the patient to clear vomit, log roll the patient with the head, neck, and trunk held in line as a unit. This can be tough to do if you are all by yourself. If you have to make a choice between a perfectly stable spine or an open airway, treat the airway. The benefits of breathing certainly outweigh the risks of spine injury.

Reduced level of consciousness (V, P, and U on the AVPU scale) can be caused by severe nervous system injury or loss of brain perfusion and oxygenation due to circulatory or respiratory system problems. There is no real way to treat a reduced level of consciousness other than to treat the cause. Basic life support is aimed at protecting the airway from fluids and vomit and the spine from further injury while assessment and treatment continues. ✚

Basic Life Support
Summary

- Treats major critical system problems
- Performed during Initial Assessment
- Precedes any non-critical treatment
- Includes:
    - CPR
    - PPV
    - Bleeding control
    - Spine stabilization

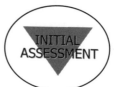

"The primary goal is to support perfusion and oxygenation of vital organs."

Chapter 4

The Circulatory System

Structure and Function

To perfuse the body tissues with oxygenated blood, the circulatory system requires adequate pumping action from the heart, an intact system of vessels, and proper vessel constriction to maintain perfusion pressure. It also requires an adequate volume of blood. To complete its part in the critical system triad, the circulatory system must have oxygen faithfully supplied to the lungs by the respiratory system, and competent nervous system control of heart rate and blood vessel pressure.

Circulatory System

Structure:
- Blood
- Vessels
- Heart

Function:
- Maintain perfusion pressure
- Circulate oxygenated blood

Problem:
- Shock: inadequate cellular oxygenation due to inadequate perfusion pressure

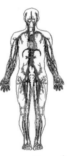

Shock

The term "shock" is often misunderstood and misrepresented. True shock is *not* caused by fatigue, disappointment, surprise, pain, grief, or any other reaction to *psychological* stress. These factors often cause acute stress reaction (ASR), which can look like shock but has none of the serious consequences.

True shock is a *physiologic* condition: the acute loss of perfusion pressure in the circulatory system resulting in inadequate perfusion and oxygenation of body cells. Shock can be the result of failure of the pumping action of the heart due to trauma or heart attack (cardiogenic shock), failure of blood vessel constriction due to anaphylaxis, infection, or spinal injury (vascular shock), or loss of circulating blood volume due to bleeding or dehydration (volume shock). True shock always indicates a life-threatening physical condition that requires specific, aggressive treatment, preferably in the hospital. Without treatment, the patient will die.

Shock

Inadequate perfusion pressure in the circulatory system

Low blood volume → Volume Shock

Poor vascular tone → Vascular Shock

Poor cardiac output → Cardiogenic Shock

"Shock is a life-threatening critical system problem requiring immediate and aggressive treatment."

Shock develops along a spectrum of severity from mild to severe. Progression can be stopped at any given point, but it is more common for shock to progress from bad to worse unless something is done about it. Of the various types of shock, the most commonly encountered in the backcountry or offshore setting is volume shock due to dehydration and, far less frequently, due to bleeding.

Volume shock is the term for inadequate pressure in the circulatory system caused by inadequate blood volume. A history of trauma sufficient to cause severe internal or external bleeding should make you think of this immediately. Typical examples include large and deep lacerations, fractures of the femur or pelvis, and blunt abdominal trauma severe enough to knock the wind out of your patient. The obvious external bleeding associated with large wounds is usually easy to find and fix. It is the internal bleeding that can be difficult to recognize and treat in the field.

Fluid loss from diarrhea, vomiting, or sweating is a more common mechanism for volume shock. Fluid can migrate between the interior of body cells, the space between the cells, and the blood itself. This ability to shift fluid explains how a patient can lose blood volume by losing water and electrolytes from sweat glands. It also explains how blood volume can be restored by *drinking* water and electrolytes.

The classic signs of volume shock, including cool and pale skin, rapid pulse, and rapid breathing, are caused by compensation mechanisms as the body attempts to maintain perfusion and oxygenation to the vital organs. The degree of change in the vital sign pattern reflects the severity of the fluid loss. The first vital sign change to occur as shock develops is shell/core effect as blood is shunted from the skin and gut into the body core. This is followed closely by an increase in the pulse and respiratory rate. If you are able to measure blood pressure, you will observe that the compensatory mechanisms will keep it near normal in the early stages.

In the long-term-care situation, measuring urine output is another good way to monitor the status of the circulatory system. Reduced blood volume will result in greatly reduced urine output as the kidneys do their part to preserve fluid. This is an important sign to watch when you're concerned about the slow loss of fluid with burns, vomiting and diarrhea, and other forms of dehydration.

Compensation may work so well that it prevents symptoms from being noticed, especially in young people. As long as the oxygenation and perfusion of the brain is adequate, your patient's level of consciousness and mental status may remain deceptively reassuring. Unless you look carefully for compensation mechanisms at work and for subtle changes in mental status, you may fail to recognize shock while there is still time to do something about it.

Compensated volume shock is not a stable condition. Unless fluid losses are stopped and volume is replaced, it will inevitably become worse. Volume shock that you cannot fix in the field deserves an emergency evacuation to definitive medical care.

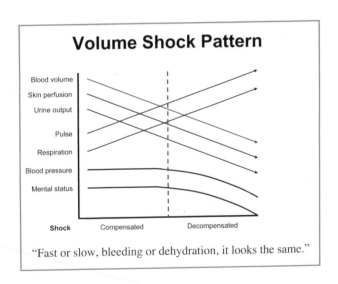

"Fast or slow, bleeding or dehydration, it looks the same."

As the compensation mechanisms are overwhelmed, oxygenation and perfusion of the brain will be impaired and the evolutionary onion will really start to peel. Mental status changes and other symptoms become more obvious as shock progresses. Ultimately, compensation will fail, perfusion pressure will fall, and level of consciousness will decay. This lethal condition is called decompensated or profound shock.

Treatment of Volume Shock: Shock from bleeding is a serious critical body system problem that you cannot treat effectively in the backcountry. The traditional "treatments" of reassurance, elevating the feet, and keeping the patient warm are certainly good for anyone in shock but do nothing to address the real problem of low blood volume. A patient in shock from severe bleeding needs replacement blood, surgeons, and a hospital. This is a true emergency and you are justified in recruiting whatever help is necessary to get the patient to the appropriate medical care. Field treatments, including intravenous fluid replacement, are just temporary measures that may help stabilize the situation long enough to reach medical care.

In the less urgent case of volume shock from slow dehydration, oral fluid replacement in the field may be sufficient if the shock is mild and you can stop the fluid losses. Oral rehydration can take some time if the patient is feeling nauseous but can be just as effective as an IV. Success will be indicated by a reversal of the volume shock pattern and the resumption of more normal urine output. If the patient continues to improve and the underlying cause of dehydration can be corrected, evacuation may not be necessary.

Volume Shock Treatment

Stop the fluid loss:
- Control bleeding
- Reduce sweating
- Treat diarrhea and vomiting

Replace fluid volume:
- IV blood and electrolyte solutions
- Oral electrolyte solutions or water and food
- Rectal or sub-cutaneous rehydration

PROP and Evacuation as Needed

Vascular shock is inadequate perfusion pressure in the circulatory system due to loss of arterial muscle tone or dilation of capillaries due to inflammation or injury. The space within the circulatory system increases with no corresponding increase in blood volume. The most common cause in the backcountry is the severe systemic allergic reaction known as anaphylaxis. Other causes include spinal cord injury, systemic infection, and the effects of some toxins.

You will see the same pattern typical in volume shock except that skin perfusion may actually be increased due to blood vessel dilation. The patient may appear flushed and red or have hives and swelling. Other signs such as fever or trauma may give you a clue to the mechanism.

Anaphylaxis can be reversed in the field with emergency medication. This treatment is covered in chapter 7, Allergy and Anaphylaxis. If the cause of vascular shock is not reversible with field treatment, as in spinal cord injury or infection, evacuation and IV fluid to expand blood volume is indicated. Keep the patient horizontal and, as with volume shock, protect him from hypothermia.

Cardiogenic shock is inadequate perfusion pressure in the circulatory system due to inadequate pumping action of the heart. The usual cause is a heart attack. Symptoms include chest pain or pressure, possibly accompanied by the signs and symptoms of shock. The pattern of compensation will resemble that of volume shock, except that the heart rate may be variable. The field treatment of a suspected heart attack is covered in chapter 20.

Cardiogenic shock from trauma is rare. It generally occurs when blood or fluid accumulates in the pericardial sack around the heart, inhibiting heart filling and reducing cardiac output. It can also develop as a result of poor function in a bruised heart. It should be suspected or anticipated whenever a trauma patient complains of persistent chest pain. Cardiogenic shock from trauma is as serious a problem as a heart attack and cannot be fixed in the field.

Acute stress reaction is not a form of shock but is worthy of mention here because of its ability to mimic the signs and symptoms of shock. Actually a nervous system problem, ASR is a frequent and normal response to physical and emotional stress of any type. ASR can coexist with real life-threatening problems, but it is more common for ASR to be a short-lived condition associated with minor injury. In fact, the victim may not even be the one injured but merely affected by the sight of another person's blood.

The use of the term "psychogenic shock" for this phenomenon can be misleading because the consequences are very different from true shock. It is important to distinguish true shock, in its various degrees of compensation and levels of severity, from an acute stress reaction, which might look similar but is not at all life threatening.

In the ambulance setting the difference is less important since both are managed as shock during the short period of treatment and transport. For long-term management in the wilderness, however, recognizing ASR for what it is can save your piece of mind and your patient from a high-risk evacuation. ASR comes in two basic forms:

Sympathetic ASR is the "speed-up" response you feel when you're anxious or scared, produced by the release of the hormone adrenalin (epinephrine). Its effect speeds up the pulse and respiratory rate, shunts blood to the muscles, dilates the pupils, and generally gets the body ready for action. It also stimulates the release of natural hormones that serve to mask the pain of injury.

This type of ASR certainly has value to human survival. It allows extraordinary efforts even in the presence of severe injury or other stress. Unfortunately, it also makes the accurate assessment of injuries difficult for the rescuer by hiding pain and altering vital signs.

Parasympathetic ASR causes fainting and nausea in response to stress, pain, or the sight of blood. It is caused by a temporary loss of perfusion of the brain due to a sudden slowing of the heart rate. The evolutionary value of this response is more difficult to figure out. This, too, is physiologically harmless except in its ability to mimic the shell/core effect seen in true volume shock and the change in mental status and vital signs seen in traumatic brain injury (TBI).

The key to recognizing acute stress reaction is in the mechanism of injury and the progression of symptoms. ASR can look like shock but can occur with or without any mechanism of injury that can cause shock. With time, ASR will get better, especially if your treatment reduces pain and anxiety. Allowing the patient to lie down, providing calm reassurance, and relieving pain by treating injuries should result in immediate improvement in symptoms.

ASR

Sympathetic:

- Mediated by epinephrine
- Increases pulse, respiration; reduces skin perfusion; increases anxiety
- Can look like shock or respiratory distress

Parasympathetic:

- Multiple chemical mediators
- Slows pulse, causes fainting
- Can look like TBI or other mechanism for mental status changes

We have all seen people with only minor extremity sprains or superficial wounds become light-headed, pale, and nauseous. Although they look "shocky," there is no cause for alarm and certainly no need for helicopters and emergency surgery. They have no mechanism for sudden volume loss.

It is important to remember that ASR can coexist with true shock. In cases where the patient has both a mechanism of injury for true shock and the signs and symptoms to go with it, you must treat it as such. The patient may later improve, revealing that most of the symptoms were due to ASR, allowing you to slow down or halt an evacuation in progress. However, if symptoms do not improve, at least you are moving in the right direction. A positive mechanism of injury and the signs and symptoms of shock is shock until proven otherwise!

▶ Case Study—Circulatory System

S: An eighteen-year-old man skiing out-of-bounds fell against a stump, injuring his right upper leg, and is unable to move without extreme pain. He reports feeling a little cold. He can feel and wiggle the toes in his right boot. He has full memory for the event and no other complaints. He denies neck or back pain or distal numbness or tingling.

The friend who reported the accident confirmed the mechanism as a direct impact to the leg. The ski patroller who found him noted that the path of his fall was about 15 feet through soft snow ending at the stump. The air temperature was 22 degrees F with a moderate north wind. It was 11:00 in the morning. All skiers in the party were accounted for.

O: Ski patrollers found the patient lying in a stable position on his back in the snow. He was shivering and uncomfortable but alert and oriented. Exam revealed a tender and swollen right thigh. There were no other major injuries found. There was no external bleeding found inside the ski clothing. Vital signs at 11:30—BP: not taken, P: 120, R: 32, C/MS: A on AVPU scale, anxious, Skin: pale and cool, T: feels cool.

A: 1. Compensated volume shock from bleeding into the thigh

A': Decompensated shock

  2. Fracture right thigh

A': Distal ischemia from artery damage or pressure

  3. Acute stress reaction

  4. Cold response

A': Hypothermia

P: 1. Immediate evacuation to a hospital and surgeon

  2. Splint thigh by immobilizing patient in a litter or toboggan

  3. Relieve pain and anxiety through treatment and reassurance

  4. Hypothermia wrap, heat packs, and transport

Discussion: This patient presents a couple of different problems common to the backcountry. He certainly has a positive mechanism for shock, and his vital sign pattern confirms it. He also has a bit of ASR, which one would expect with a broken leg. The cold environment and immobility of the patient adds the *anticipated* problem of hypothermia. ✚

Shock
Wilderness Context
High-Risk Problem:

- Cannot stop fluid loss
- Cannot replace fluids
- Persistent chest pain
- Coexisting major problems
- Cannot maintain body core temperature
- Persistent s/sx of shock despite treatment

These cases may be worth a high risk evacuation or an attempt to bring advanced level care to the patient.

Chapter 5

The Respiratory System

Structure and Function

One of the critical body systems, the respiratory system performs the task of bringing oxygen to the blood and removing carbon dioxide. The exchange takes place in the alveoli of the lungs, where only a thin, semipermeable membrane separates the outside air from the blood. The rest of the system consists of semirigid tubes to conduct air to the alveoli, and a bellows system composed of the chest wall and muscles for moving the air in and out.

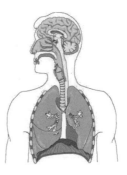

Respiratory System

Structure:
- Upper airway
- Lower airway
- Alveoli
- Chest Wall and Diaphragm
- Neuro drive

Function:
- Oxygenation of the blood
- Regulation of blood pH

Problem:
- Respiratory distress, failure, and arrest

Like the circulatory system, the respiratory system is under nervous system control. In a healthy patient, breathing is controlled by the brain as it measures the pH (acidity) of the blood. This is actually a reflection of the amount of dissolved carbon dioxide. Too much CO_2 in the blood causes the acidity to increase. The brain responds by increasing the rate and depth of respiration to "blow off" the CO_2 until a normal pH is reestablished. Conversely, too little CO_2 is corrected by decreasing the rate and depth of respiration.

This CO_2 regulation system is very precise and results in a smooth and regular respiratory pattern. But in some disease conditions, such as emphysema, the amount of CO_2 in the blood is high all the time because the lungs are damaged and cannot function properly. The brain then falls back on measuring the amount of oxygen in the blood to determine breathing rate and depth. This is much less precise, is more easily upset, and results in a more irregular pattern.

As with the circulatory system, we try to reduce the respiratory system to its simplest component parts. Knowing this basic anatomy will help you determine what type of problem your patient might be experiencing and what might be done to treat it:

FIVE BASIC COMPONENTS

1. Upper Airway—Consists of the mouth (oropharynx), nose (nasopharynx), and throat (larynx).

2. Lower Airway—Composed of large tubes (trachea), smaller tubes (bronchi), and the smallest tubes (bronchioles).

3. Alveoli—The membranous air sacks at the end of the system adjacent to blood-filled capillaries, where oxygen and carbon dioxide exchange occurs.

4. Chest Wall/Diaphragm—In normal function inspiration (the intake of air) is caused by the active contraction of the diaphragm and chest wall muscles, which expand the chest cavity, sucking air into the lungs. Expiration (air out) is a passive process that occurs when these muscles relax and the natural elasticity of the lungs and chest squeeze the air out.

5. Nervous System Control—The nervous system (brain) controls the rate and depth of respiration in response to the amount of carbon dioxide and oxygen in the blood.

Respiratory Distress, Failure, and Arrest

Respiratory distress is the generic term for dozens of different problems that can develop directly in the respiratory system or as the indirect result of circulatory or nervous system problems. They usually produce the same generic symptoms, including increased respiratory rate, increased effort, and unusual noise like wheezing, cough, or the stuttering inhalation against an obstruction known as "stridor." All have the same generic effect: reduced oxygen supply to the blood.

One of the most obvious signs of respiratory distress is the use of accessory muscles. Normally, a person at rest uses only the diaphragm to breathe. When work is increased, oxygen demand increases and the respiratory system will use muscles in the chest, shoulders, and neck to increase the depth of respiration. You would expect to see this as a normal response in someone who is running or hiking hard. You would not expect to see it in someone sitting still. Accessory muscle use at rest indicates respiratory distress.

A more subtle sign is shortness of breath on exertion. This patient has a compromised respiratory system that is capable of supplying enough oxygen only if the demand is low. Sitting and resting are fine, but walking causes severe shortness of breath. This symptom is often an early sign of respiratory distress due to pneumonia, high altitude pulmonary edema, or asthma.

Whatever the cause of respiratory distress, it will progress to respiratory failure if it is not corrected. An ominous sign is the inability to speak more than a few words between breaths. This is called one- or two-word dyspnea. A patient in this condition is in serious trouble. Conversely, a patient who is able to talk at length about their shortness of breath is probably okay for now.

Failure means that the respiratory system cannot supply enough oxygen to the blood to keep the brain functioning normally. The primary indicator is decay in mental status and level of consciousness. If not corrected, the inevitable result will be respiratory arrest.

Respiratory distress that you cannot fix in the field is a life-threatening problem. The progression to failure may be rapid or slow. The treatment and evacuation may be a desperate emergency or a careful and low-stress process. The generic problem is the same, but the specific treatment is determined by the severity and rate of progression and by the part of the respiratory system that is involved.

Respiratory Problems

Respiratory Distress:
- Difficulty breathing, speaks in short sentences.
- A on AVPU, anxious

Respiratory Failure:
- Able to speak only one or two words at a time.
- A, lethargic to V, or P on AVPU

Respiratory Arrest:
- No breathing
- U on AVPU

Respiratory distress is one of the most frightening problems that you will ever deal with in field medicine. Having an automatic response to the immediate problem should get treatment going while you calm yourself and develop a more specific assessment and plan. This generic treatment for respiratory distress is abbreviated PROP.

Generic Treatment for Respiratory Distress: PROP

Position—Any patient in respiratory distress who is able to move will have already found the best position in which to breathe. This is usually sitting up to allow gravity to assist the diaphragm and to help keep fluids out of the airway tubes. In unconscious or immobile patients, special care must be taken to position them in a way that prevents airway obstruction from secretions, vomit, or the collapse of their own airway. This is usually on their side, with the head and neck in the "in line" position.

Reassurance—Encourage the patient to breathe slower and deeper rather than panting like a dog. This brings in fresh oxygen rather than moving the same old carbon dioxide back and forth in the tubes.

Oxygen—If available, giving supplemental oxygen will increase the concentration of oxygen getting into the blood and, ultimately, to the brain.

Positive Pressure Ventilation—A patient in respiratory distress will fatigue rapidly. You might need to provide positive pressure ventilation to assist the patient's efforts. This PPV produced by the rescuer blowing air in as the patient tries to inhale can often work where the patient cannot draw air in on his or her own.

More specific treatment for respiratory distress will depend on which part of the respiratory system is affected. Identifying the location and type of respiratory system problem is the goal of your initial assessment and focused history and exam. Although both you and your patient will be distracted by ASR, you must make an attempt to identify and treat the specific cause if at all possible.

Specific Treatments for Respiratory Distress
UPPER AIRWAY OBSTRUCTION

The upper airway may be obstructed by the tongue, a piece of food, or the fact that the patient's head is under water. Obstruction can also develop slowly with the swelling from trauma or infection. If the initial assessment reveals the absence of respiration, even if the patient is still conscious, Basic Life Support including airway opening maneuvers must begin immediately (see chapter 3, Basic Life Support).

If airway obstruction is not complete, the patient may have noisy and difficult respiration. The term "stridor" is used to describe the stuttering sound made by inhalation against an upper airway obstruction. The ability to swallow is often impaired, and the patient may be drooling. Talking may be difficult or impossible.

The important question in treating a partial obstruction in the field is whether the patient is getting enough air to support brain function until medical care can be reached. Look for signs that oxygenation of the blood is adequate: good skin color, A on the AVPU scale, and no worsening of the respiratory distress.

Treatment of Upper Airway Obstruction: For the treatment of respiratory arrest or failure due to airway obstruction, or partial obstruction with inadequate oxygenation, refer to Basic Life Support (chapter 3). In cases where a foreign object is lodged in the throat for a brief time and successfully removed before the patient gets in trouble, you may certainly congratulate yourself on a real "save." However, the object may have caused enough irritation of the airway to result in the development of obstruction from swelling later on, and this should be on your anticipated problem list for the next twenty-four hours.

In cases of partial airway obstruction with respiratory distress but no signs of failure, the rule is "do no harm." Apply the generic treatment for respiratory distress and evacuate quickly. In almost all cases of partial obstruction, breathing cool air will reduce swelling of the airway temporarily. Be prepared to perform airway opening maneuvers if it becomes apparent that the airway is closing. A partial obstruction frequently becomes worse over time.

Upper Airway Obstruction

MOI:	Assessment:	Treatment:
Cork	Incomplete	PROP
Kink	resp distress	BLS:
Fluids	whistling	reposition airway
Swelling	stridor	remove obstruction
Epiglottis	Complete	ALS:
Anaphylaxis	resp arrest	surgical airway
	silence	medications
	choking signs	*epinephrine*
		diphenhyramine
		prednisone

"With a partial obstruction, the first rule of treatment is, Do no harm."

LOWER AIRWAY CONSTRICTION

Spasm, swelling, or the accumulation of mucus or pus can cause narrowing of the lower airway tubes (bronchi and bronchioles). This is what happens in asthma, bronchitis, and anaphylaxis. The effect is to slow the movement of air in and out of the alveoli. Expiration is often prolonged, with wheezing and gurgling. Sometimes, the lower airway noise is loud enough to hear from a distance. Other times you may need a stethoscope or an ear to the patient's chest.

The patient may describe exposure to smoke, inhaled water, or other irritating substance indicating a generalized swelling. He may have been exposed to something to which he is allergic, indicating anaphylaxis. Or there may be a history of slowly worsening illness and fever pointing to respiratory infection. Whatever the cause, the patient usually develops a cough as the respiratory system tries to clear itself. There may be an obvious increase in respiratory effort as the system struggles to move air against increased resistance. Vital signs may show the use of compensatory mechanisms with elevated heart and respiratory rate.

Treatment of Lower Airway Constriction: Beyond PROP, the specific treatment for lower airway constriction includes antibiotics for infection and inhaled medications to dilate the bronchial tubes for asthma. Severe respiratory distress from these conditions will not respond well to simple PROP. Anaphylaxis and severe asthma can be treated on an emergency basis with injectable epinephrine. The treatment of these conditions are covered in chapters 7 and 8.

Lower Airway Constriction

MOI:	Assessment:	Treatment:
Swelling	Resp Distress	PROP
Spasm	wheezing	ALS:
Asthma	cough	intubation
Anaphylaxis	History	medications
Bronchitis	exposure	*epinephrine*
Burns	*asthma*	*albuterol*
	allergy	*prednisone*
	illness	

"The ideal treatment is medication to relieve the constriction and treat the cause."

PULMONARY EDEMA

Excess fluid that accumulates in the alveoli, blocking the exchange of oxygen and carbon dioxide between air and blood, is called pulmonary edema. This fluid usually comes from within the body as capillaries leak into the alveoli. This can be the result of too much pressure in the pulmonary part of the circulatory system, as in congestive heart failure, or swelling in reaction to irritants such as water or smoke. It can also be an effect of reduced oxygen at high altitude. Contusion or laceration of the lung tissue may cause the alveoli to fill with blood. Pneumonia is pulmonary edema from infection.

Large amounts of fluid in the lungs will cause gurgling, which can be heard at a distance. Fluid may actually froth at the mouth. Small amounts of fluid may be heard with a stethoscope or an ear to the chest as "crackling" on respiration. Vital signs will show that the body is compensating for partial loss of lung function with an increase in respiratory and pulse rates. The development of fever indicates infection.

In less severe cases this reduced lung function may not be noticeable until the patient exerts himself. With the increased demands of exercise, the reduced lung capacity will become obvious as the patient becomes short of breath much more easily than would be normal for him. This shortness of breath on exertion is an early form of respiratory distress. Coughing is common with the onset of more significant pulmonary edema.

Treatment of Pulmonary Edema: PROP may make a significant difference here. Like most patients in respiratory distress, the patient will prefer to sit up even during litter evacuation. In severe cases of pulmonary edema with respiratory failure, positive pressure ventilation can force fluid out of the alveoli and open more area for gas exchange. Specific treatments include antibiotics for pneumonia, medications and descent for high-altitude pulmonary edema, and medications to reduce fluid load and improve heart function load in cardiogenic pulmonary edema.

Pulmonary Edema

MOI:	Assessment:	Treatment:
Smoke	Resp Distress	PROP
Drowning	cough	ALS:
Infection	crackles	intubation
Lung contusion	gurgling	medications
pneumonia	frothy sputum	diuretics
HAPE	History	steroids
CHF	exposure	antibiotics
ARDS	altitude	nifedipine
	illness	

"Positive pressure ventilation can help force alveolar fluid back into the circulatory system, restoring lung surface area for gas exchange."

CHEST TRAUMA

Trauma to the chest wall or airway tubes can interfere with the function of the respiratory system in a number of ways. Chest trauma with persistent respiratory distress is best evacuated without delay. The injuries are often complicated and severe and cannot be effectively managed in the field.

You should look carefully for bruising and deformity and palpate for fractured ribs. An unstable chest wall, also called a "flail chest," indicates that the bellows system is damaged to the point that it is no longer rigid. Instead of the lungs expanding equally with inspiration, part of the chest wall collapses inward.

Hemothorax and pneumothorax are terms used to describe the presence of blood or air in the space between the lungs and the chest wall, preventing full expansion of the lungs and putting pressure on the heart and large blood vessels in the chest. In the case of an open pneumothorax, sometimes called a "sucking chest wound," air may enter the chest cavity through an injury in the chest wall. In a closed pneumothorax, air may enter the chest cavity through an injured lung. It may affect only one side or both.

Signs of hemo- or pneumothorax include increasing respiratory distress and chest pain. In the early stages or in mild cases, there may be no outward signs. In severe cases you may see increased expansion of the chest on one side or deviation of the trachea in the neck away from the side of the pneumothorax. Any obvious chest wall deformity, tracheal deviation, or unequal expansion of the lungs indicates a severe life-threatening respiratory problem.

In less severe trauma, where only one or two ribs may be fractured, most of the patient's respiratory distress will probably be due to pain. This inhibits deep inspiration, causing the patient to breathe in shallow, quick breaths. Acute stress reaction may also be a major component of the patient's discomfort.

Treatment of Chest Trauma: PROP is limited in effect and temporary only. The patient with chest injury significant enough to cause respiratory distress deserves immediate evacuation to surgical care. A patient who can move will naturally find the best position in which to breathe. This is usually sitting up. If the patient with chest wall trauma prefers to lie down, position him on the injured side to help splint the chest wall and help keep blood from building up in the uninjured side of the chest.

In cases of open chest wounds with air passing in and out of the hole, the injury should be covered with an airtight seal such as a piece of plastic bag. Don't worry about trying to make a one-way valve or coordinating the patch placement with inspiration. Just put it on. If applying a patch improves the situation, leave it in place. If symptoms become worse, remove it.

In case of a simple rib fracture, reducing pain by finding a comfortable position and using pain medication will make breathing more comfortable and reduce respiratory distress. A rib belt wrapped around the chest sometimes helps in pain control and allows for easier respiration. It may also tend to restrict breathing and make the situation worse. If a belt is applied, pay attention to the patient and the respiratory status and be prepared to adjust or remove it.

Chest Wall Trauma

MOI:
Puncture
Rib Fracture
Diaphragm
  rupture
Spontaneous
  pneumothorax

Assessment:
Resp Distress
cough
crepitis
trachial shift
deformity
bloody sputum
breath sounds

Treatment:
PROP
BLS:
  patch the leaks
  splint chest
ALS:
  intubation
  chest decompression
  pain medication

"The patient with chest injury significant enough to cause respiratory distress deserves immediate evacuation."

DECREASED NERVOUS SYSTEM DRIVE: HYPOVENTILATION

If brain function is impaired by low blood sugar, hypothermia, hypoxia, or any other problem, respiratory effort may be irregular or slow. The symptoms are a marked contrast to the other forms of respiratory distress. Where problems like asthma and chest wall trauma tend to cause noisy and dramatic symptoms and ASR, respiratory failure from loss of nervous system control is usually very quiet. The fact that respiration is inadequate is not always clear.

The level of consciousness will already be reduced by whatever is causing the primary nervous system problem and is not a good indicator. You may see cyanosis (blue lips and skin) or realize that the respiratory rate and depth is well below normal. To be safe, anyone with slowed or irregular breathing and reduced consciousness should be considered in need of positive pressure ventilation and oxygen. Don't be timid about this; PPV carries a very low risk of causing harm and great benefit if the patient really needs it.

Treatment for Hypoventilation: PROP includes PPV and positioning or careful monitoring to avoid airway obstruction by the tongue. These patients are also at risk for aspirating vomit, saliva, or blood into the lungs. Aspiration of vomit carries a very high mortality rate and must be avoided at all costs. In any patient with altered level of consciousness, vomiting and airway obstruction is on the anticipated problem list. If the airway cannot be continuously monitored and protected, the patient should be positioned to allow for drainage from the mouth and nose. Urgent evacuation is indicated unless the underlying nervous system problem can be corrected in the field.

INCREASED NERVOUS SYSTEM DRIVE: HYPERVENTILATION

Increased respiratory drive occurs with altitude, exercise, injury, and illness. This is a normal response to physiologic demands requiring more oxygen and producing more carbon dioxide. Increased respiration also occurs with acute stress reaction but not in response to an increased need. The result of hyperventilation in ASR can be an abnormal *decrease* in the carbon dioxide concentration in the blood with the associated abnormal decrease in acidity. This is blood chemistry out of balance, which can produce a variety of nervous system symptoms that are referred to as "hyperventilation syndrome."

Hyperventilation can occur with or without obvious fast and heavy breathing. It only takes a slight increase in depth and rate over time to cause changes in blood acidity. The respiratory changes observed in your measurement of vital signs may be very subtle. It can be difficult to distinguish between hyperventilation syndrome and other nervous system problems, especially if there is a positive mechanism for injury. As with other components of ASR, it gets better with time and basic treatment.

There are some classic nervous system effects of hyperventilation syndrome worth mentioning. Tingling of the hands and feet and numbness around the mouth is common. The patient may feel paralyzed, but their ability to move is not actually impaired. The patient may report that they see black spots or a narrowing of the visual fields.

Treatment of Hyperventilation: PROP is part of the treatment, primarily in reassuring the patient that the condition is not serious. Telling the patient that hyperventilation is causing their symptoms almost always cures it. Coach the patient to breathe slower. If this does not improve the situation, take another look for causes other than ASR.

The popular home remedy of having the patient breathe into a paper bag will have the effect of increasing the carbon dioxide in the blood. But it will also have the effect of decreasing the oxygen supply. This is neither safe nor effective.

▶ Case Study—Respiratory System

A backcountry ranger responded to the scene of an apparent illness on the Raquette Falls portage. It was mid-morning, the weather was partly cloudy with light winds and temperatures in the 60s. One member of a group of twelve teenagers was having trouble breathing. The rest of the group was accounted for and in no trouble.

S: A thirteen-year-old boy with a history of asthma developed respiratory distress in the middle of a mile-long portage. Witnesses reported that he used his medication inhaler just before setting out but soon became short of breath. He set his canoe on a tree and slumped to the ground, having trouble catching his breath. There was no history of trauma or insect stings. The boy had no allergies. He was taking no additional medications. Asthma had been diagnosed several years ago. He last ate at 0900. He had not been otherwise ill.

O: Initial assessment showed an awake and anxious boy in obvious respiratory distress. Exam revealed no other injury. Vital signs at 1100 were: P: 120, R: 40 with wheezing, BP: not obtained, S: cool, pale, blue lips, T: felt cool, but core temperature probably okay, C/MS: Awake, but anxious

A: Respiratory distress from lower airway constriction (asthma)

A': Respiratory failure

P: The boy was assisted into a sitting position to help breathing. Group members were sent to both ends of the portage to look for the boy's medication. Oxygen was not available, but the ranger was carrying a pocket mask to use for PPV if necessary.

The asthma inhaler was never found. Evacuation was carried out by canoe to an ALS ambulance crew that had been called by radio. By the end of the trip, the patient was V on AVPU, and positive pressure ventilation had been started. Following treatment in the ambulance and hospital, the boy improved quickly.

Discussion: With the history available from group members, the ranger could make the specific assessment of asthma and include the boy's medication in the plan. Without this information, he would be left with the general diagnosis of respiratory distress due to lower airway constriction. There could be several causes, but the treatment would be the same. Had the ranger been trained in the use of injectable epinephrine for severe asthma, this emergency treatment could have been initiated in the field. ✚

Respiratory Distress
Wilderness Context

High-Risk Problem:

- Cannot improve respiratory status
- Persistent altered mental status
- Coexisting major problems
- Cyanosis
- Cannot maintain body core temperature
- Cannot maintain hydration and calories
- The patient is getting worse

Chapter 6

The Nervous System

Structure and Function

The nervous system consists of the brain, spinal cord, and peripheral nerves. The brain, in addition to being responsible for remembering where you left your flashlight, controls all critical life functions. Its primary connection with the circulatory and respiratory systems is through the spinal cord. Both the brain and cord are encased and protected within the bony structure of the skull and vertebrae of the spine.

From the gap between vertebrae, peripheral nerves branch out from the spinal cord to all body tissues. Nerves controlling the most critical functions exit the cord at the base of the skull and in the neck. This is why spinal cord injuries that occur in this area can cause extreme disability or death due to the loss of nervous system control over vital body functions.

All nervous system tissue is extremely sensitive to injury, especially oxygen deprivation. If the brain is involved, reduced oxygenation and perfusion will immediately affect mental status, giving one of the best first indicators of a developing life-threatening condition. This is what we like to call "peeling the evolutionary onion."

Central Nervous System
Brain

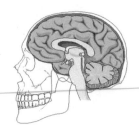

Structure:

- Cerebrum
- Cerebellum
- Brain stem
- Cerebrospinal fluid

Function:

- Voluntary Action
- Involuntary Control

Problem:

- Impaired brain function

For field purposes we describe brain function by using a scale abbreviated AVPU. This simple assessment tool is familiar to most emergency care providers. A common notation for this assessment is Consciousness and Mental Status, abbreviated C/MS.

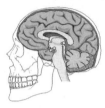
In describing mental status, plain language is usually best. Describing your patient as "awake, knows his name and where he is, but not sure how he got here or what day of the week it is" may seem cumbersome, but everyone involved in his care and transport will understand it. Furthermore, improvement or decay in mental status will be more easily detected and described. The numerous causes of impaired brain function can be summarized with the simple mnemonic **STOPEATS:**

S–Sugar: blood sugar, low or high
T–Temperature: hypothermia or hyperthermia
O–Oxygen: hypoxia from suffocation
P–Pressure: increased intracranial pressure from brain injury
E–Electricity: household current or lightning
A–Altitude: hypoxia from HAPE, pressure from HAPE
T–Toxins: drugs, poisons, intoxicants
S–Salts: electrolyte imbalance such as exertional hyponatremia

STOPEATS can be a handy diagnostic tool when you are seeing changes in mental status or level of consciousness and you are not sure what is causing it. You will usually be able to eliminate some possible causes in your survey of the scene and examination of the patient. Other possibilities will have to remain on your problem list until they can be ruled out or confirmed over time.

Imagine caring for the subject of a successful forty-eight-hour backcountry search. Your patient is found curled up under a spruce tree in a level area of forest at 950 meters in elevation. The weather is cool and wet without thunderstorm activity. He is V on the APVU scale and shivering. There is no evidence of injury.

Already you can eliminate problems with pressure, electricity, oxygen, and altitude from your problem list. Even though you are fairly certain that his problem is hypothermia, the mnemonic reminds you to consider blood sugar, toxins, and salts as possible contributing factors. Time and response to treatment may allow you to further refine your problem list in the field, or you may have to keep a potential problem on the list throughout an evacuation effort. Treat what you can, and evacuate for what you can't.

Impaired Brain Function

Mechanisms:

S – Sugar

T – Temperature

O – Oxygen

P – Pressure

E – Electricity

A – Altitude

T – Toxins

S – Salts

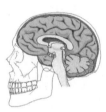

"The numerous causes of impaired brain function can be summarized … with the mnemonic *STOPEATS*."

Increased Intracranial Pressure

This is the "P" in the STOPEATS mnemonic and the brain problem that is most likely to be fatal. The brain, like other body tissues, will swell from bleeding and edema when injured. Unlike other tissues the brain is confined within the rigid structure of the skull, where there simply is not much additional space. Swelling within the skull can produce a dangerous rise in intracranial pressure, which can become severe enough to prevent perfusion and oxygenation of brain tissue. Common causes include traumatic brain injury, stroke, high-altitude cerebral edema, heat stroke, and prolonged hypoxia such as in near-drowning events.

Like volume shock, increased ICP has a typical pattern and spectrum of severity regardless of its cause or rate of onset. Although other vital sign changes occur, altered mental status ("peeling the onion") is often the earliest vital sign indicator of increasing ICP. The patient may be disoriented or appear "drunk," combative, or restless. These signs will typically be accompanied by severe headache, photophobia, and nausea.

If the pressure continues to increase, the deeper layers of brain function will begin to show the effects with the onset of vomiting and a severe headache. The cerebral edema and pressure may or may not get worse, but you will now be very concerned about that possibility. Vomiting also adds the anticipated problems of airway obstruction and dehydration.

Symptoms of severe increased ICP include a decrease in the level of consciousness with seizures, posturing, and pupil dilation as the brain stem is pressed against the floor of the cranium. At this point, survival without neurosurgical intervention is unlikely. In the ideal situation, any patient with increased ICP as an anticipated problem is evacuated from the field *before* it develops.

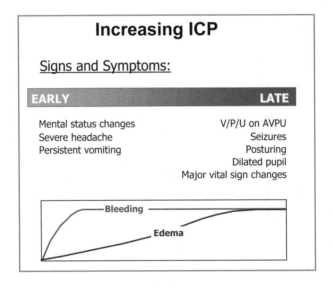

Treatment of Increased ICP: The rapid onset of severe swelling from traumatic brain injury will be fatal in most backcountry or offshore situations. Cardiorespiratory arrest due to severe brain damage does not respond to CPR or defibrillation. It is the early recognition of slow-onset swelling from less severe trauma or other causes that can save lives in the wilderness setting. The appropriate response is good Basic Life Support and urgent evacuation.

There is no field treatment specific to increased intracranial pressure that will improve survival. However, your careful attention to airway control, ventilation, preservation of body core temperature, and hydration can certainly improve the outcome. Evacuation to surgical care is a priority, but support of vital body functions during the evacuation is equally essential.

Increased ICP

Field Treatment:

- Urgent evacuation to neurosurgical care

- Emergency descent or Gamow bag for AMS

- Maintain body core temperature

- Maintain hydration and calories

- Maintain airway, PROP

- Stabilize spine:
    - if spine cannot be cleared
    - if stabilization will not increase risk

Traumatic Brain Injury

Traumatic brain injury (TBI) is the common term for brain damage from trauma. The term "head injury" is also commonly used but can be confused with injuries to the face or soft tissue that may or may not include brain injury. TBI is diagnosed in the field by observing or obtaining a history of a change in brain function at the time of injury. The change may be as dramatic as a ten-minute loss of consciousness or as subtle as a brief loss of memory or short period of feeling confused and disoriented.

Any traumatic brain injury carries the anticipated problem (A') of increased ICP. Generally, the more severe the injury the more likely the brain is to swell. A mild injury would be indicated by a very brief loss of consciousness or a loss of memory for the event only. Severe injury is evidenced by profound and prolonged changes in mental status, loss of memory for the hours before the event, or persistent lapses of memory after the event.

One real advantage of being able to diagnose TBI in the field is being able to determine when a patient doesn't have one. Injuries to the face and scalp without a change in brain function do not carry the A' of increased ICP. There may be an ugly scalp laceration or a broken nose, but if the patient remembers everything that happened, there is no brain injury. Remember: At sea, as in the mountains, it is just as important to know when you don't have a medical emergency as when you do.

When TBI *is* on the problem list, the important question becomes whether the injured brain tissue will swell enough to cause a dangerous increase in intracranial pressure. This is a common backcountry medical dilemma. Evacuate now, or wait and watch?

The answer is easy when the level of consciousness remains severely altered. Immediate emergency evacuation is ideal. Even with minor TBI, medical evaluation is a good idea when the risk of evacuation is minimal. Increased ICP is a serious critical system problem, and its presence on your anticipated problem list, however unlikely, is of real concern.

The decision becomes more difficult when your evacuation options present significant risk. There are no absolute rules to fit every situation, but there are some general guidelines to help with your risk/benefit assessment. Generally, there is a higher probability of increasing ICP when brain function does not return to normal shortly after the event. Persistent disorientation or the inability to retain new memory is an ominous sign. The patient may literally forget what has been happening from minute to minute as you talk to them. This is sometimes referred to as anterograde amnesia.

Amnesia for a significant time period is another cause for concern. This is the snowboarder who struck his head and now doesn't know where he is, how he came to be there, or with whom. He may not know the month or time of year. This indicates a more severe brain injury than the patient who does not remember the accident itself but remembers everything else.

A history of previous TBI is also worrisome, especially if it was within the past few weeks. Incompletely healed brain tissue is prone to swelling, and scar tissue is more prone to bleeding. To get an idea how severe a previous brain injury might have been, ask if the patient was hospitalized.

Evidence of skull fracture tells you that your patient has sustained a significant impact. The potential for bleeding and swelling is increased. The patient is also at risk for infection over the long term.

Traumatic Brain Injury
Wilderness Context

<u>High-Risk Problem:</u>

- Persistent disorientation
- Cannot retain new memory
- History of recent previous TBI
- Skull fracture
- High velocity or high mass impact
- S/sx of increased ICP

"Generally, the more severe the injury, the more likely the brain is to swell."

Treatment of Traumatic Brain Injury: TBI requires no specific field treatment. However, it is important to monitor the patient carefully for at least twenty-four hours to detect the onset of increased ICP. Patients being monitored should not use narcotic or stimulant drugs or drink alcohol since this will confuse the assessment of the level of consciousness and mental status. It is not necessary to keep the patient awake. The pain and vomiting of increasing ICP will wake them if necessary.

Generally, in a remote backcountry setting it is best to begin planning for the evacuation of a patient with confirmed TBI rather than wait for the onset of increasing ICP. This is especially true of patients with more significant signs and symptoms. We also must remember to evaluate and treat for spine injury, which has the same mechanism of injury.

Post Concussive Syndrome

Following a blow to the head, some patients experience symptoms including headache, photophobia, insomnia, or sleep disturbance developing more than twenty-four hours after the injury. This can occur with or without TBI. This post concussive syndrome does not indicate increasing ICP and may be observed and treated symptomatically.

The symptoms of post concussive syndrome can be expected to wax and wane and may persist for days or weeks. Generally, nonurgent medical follow-up is adequate. However, progressive worsening or the appearance of new symptoms should motivate urgent evacuation and early medical evaluation.

Stroke

A stroke is what the medical profession politely refers to as a "cerebral vascular accident," as if the brain didn't really mean to do it. The accident happens when a blood vessel inside the brain ruptures and bleeds, or a clot lodges in an artery. The initial effect of either event is ischemia and infarction, which may be localized or very extensive. Elevated ICP may soon follow, especially with intracranial bleeding.

A sudden change in brain function without a history of trauma or intoxication should make you think of stroke. It may be as subtle as a little numbness in one hand or arm or a slight facial droop, or as dramatic as complete paralysis of one side of the body or the sudden loss of the ability to speak. In some cases the symptoms are transient, resolving after a few minutes or hours as a clot forms and then dissolves. These "transient ischemic attacks" are a warning of serious trouble to come.

Like a heart attack, a stroke is an example of ischemia to infarction in a critical body system, and it is a life-threatening problem. The patient needs a hospital. Apply basic life support and treat as you would any patient with existing or anticipated increased ICP and initiate an emergency evacuation. Do not give aspirin or ibuprofen in an effort to reduce clotting. The problem may actually be caused by bleeding and you will have no way of knowing that in the field.

Seizures

Brain tissue has electrical properties much like heart tissue. Seizures are caused by an uncoordinated burst of electrical activity in the brain. They have a variety of causes. The important consideration in assessment is the context in which the seizure occurs. Seizures can be part of the pattern of increased ICP in trauma patients or a relatively normal occurrence in a patient with epilepsy. They can be related to drug use, heat stroke, or any of the other mechanisms summarized in the STOPEATS mnemonic. Seizure can also occur for no apparent reason in an otherwise healthy individual.

The classic grand mal seizure is characterized by generalized tensing of all body muscles and repetitive, purposeless movement. Although the eyes may be open, the patient will be unresponsive during the seizure. He may be incontinent of feces and urine. There will usually be a period of drowsiness and disorientation after the seizure has ended.

Seizure
Wilderness Context

High Risk Problem:

- Result of trauma or environmental illness
- Persistent neurological deficit
- New onset seizure
- Recurrent or persistent seizure
- The patient is getting worse

"The real worry, of course, is not the seizure itself but what may have caused it."

Treatment of Seizure: Protection from injury is the most important treatment that you can provide. Most seizures will resolve spontaneously in a short period of time. Protect the patient from injury when falling or thrashing. Protect the patient from unnecessary treatments, such as chest compressions or rescuers trying to force objects between their teeth.

Seizing patients will normally hold their breath briefly and become cyanotic. This is not a problem as long as it does not last more than a couple of minutes. Position the patient and ventilate if necessary after the seizure has resolved or during the seizure if you feel that respirations are inadequate.

The real worry, of course, is not the seizure itself but what has caused it. Unless the patient is a known epileptic who has frequent seizures, the cause must be researched by a medical practitioner. Because the seizure may be the first sign of a serious condition, evacuation is a good idea. If the seizure resolves spontaneously and the patient seems otherwise okay, this is not an emergency.

Intoxication

Intoxication refers to a change in brain function due to the effects of a foreign chemical, often intentional. This is the second "T" in STOPEATS. Alcohol and narcotics are common examples, but there are hundreds of others. For emergency work the effects can be generally classified as depressant or stimulant. Depressants are the most dangerous, especially when they reduce the nervous system control of respiratory drive.

Your survey of the scene and history should clue you in to the mechanism of injury. If the intoxication is severe, with the patient below V on the AVPU scale, the patient will be at risk for airway obstruction and inadequate respiration. In less severe cases the danger may be indirect, such as hypothermia, frostbite, or stumbling overboard.

Treatment of Intoxication: Protect the airway from vomit, fluids, or mechanical obstruction. Give positive pressure ventilation if respiration seems inadequate. Protect the patient from heat loss. Evacuate if the patient is not improving. Fortunately, most intoxicating chemicals will be metabolized and excreted by the body within a few hours.

▶ Case Study—Nervous System

A forty-year-old fisherman was struck on the head while trying to secure a trawl door on a 47-foot fishing vessel 50 miles offshore. The time was 0430. The weather was clear with winds of 15 knots, a sea of 3 feet, and temperature in the 20s with light freezing spray.

S: This patient was found face down on deck within seconds of being seen upright at the rail. The unsecured gear was clear of the scene and the patient's position was momentarily stable.

O: He was breathing and U on the AVPU scale for about two minutes before beginning to respond to questions. Once he was secure below decks, further exam showed swelling and discoloration on the back of his head but no other injury. He complained of headache and vomited twice. Vital signs at 0500: P: 60, R: 12, BP: 140/72, S: warm, dry, T: 97.0 rectally, C/MS: V on AVPU

A: Head injury (concussion)

A': 1. Elevated ICP

    2. Airway obstruction from vomit

P: Cervical collar, secured in litter, wrapped to prevent heat loss. Fishing gear secured, Coast Guard notified, and the vessel under way for the nearest port. Airway constantly monitored.

Discussion: This is a nice, neat case for evacuation. The patient's signs and symptoms fit the red flags for head injury. The patient was carefully monitored for signs of increasing ICP and any threat to the airway. The possibility of a helicopter evacuation was discussed with the Coast Guard, but the patient remained stable and did not vomit again. He arrived in port without incident. ✚

Chapter 7
Allergy and Anaphylaxis

The severe systemic allergic reaction known as anaphylaxis is a major problem affecting all three critical systems. The use of the medication for immediate field treatment is now considered part of basic life support. The procedure is especially important to people traveling out of range of the emergency medical services. Anaphylaxis is a problem that will not wait for an ambulance or helicopter to arrive.

Allergy is an abnormal immune system response to contact with a foreign substance known as an antigen. Examples of antigens include bee venom, peanut oil, and penicillin. Actually, almost anything can be an antigen. It is interesting to note that a significant percentage of the patients who present to emergency departments with severe allergic reactions don't know exactly what they are allergic to.

The immune response results in the release of excess amounts of the chemical histamine into blood and body tissues. Histamine dilates the blood vessels and constricts the lower airways. These effects can be mild or severe, local or systemic. Onset can be nearly instantaneous or delayed by several hours.

When the response remains localized to the area of antigen contact, it is called a local reaction. The patient experiences swelling, itching, and redness from dilation of blood vessels. Hay fever is an example of a local reaction affecting the mucous membranes of the nose and eyes. Poison ivy produces a local allergic reaction on the skin surface.

Allergy and Anaphylaxis

Mechanism:

- Antigen injected, ingested, inhaled, or absorbed

- Antibody produced by the immune system marking the antigen for destruction by white blood cells

- Histamine released by white blood cells during the process

Anaphylaxis

Signs and Symptoms:

- Generalized hives, itching, swelling
- Tight or scratchy throat
- Vascular and volume shock
- Respiratory distress
- Nausea, vomiting, diarrhea
- Altered mental status

| Local reaction | Mild Allergic Reaction | Anaphylaxis |

Anaphylaxis, by contrast, is a system-wide allergic reaction produced when large amounts of histamine are released into the general circulation. Hives, swelling, and itching develop throughout the body. The patient may give a history of a specific allergy, or the history may be completely unrevealing.

In its mild form it is characterized by generalized itching and hives with no swelling, no respiratory involvement, and no signs of shock. This mild allergic reaction often resolves on its own or responds well to treatment with non-prescription antihistamines such as diphenhydramine. Often, the patient will give a history of similar symptoms and successful treatment with oral medications. This is reassuring for field treatment but still requires careful monitoring because any reaction can be more severe than expected.

Severe anaphylaxis, also called anaphylactic shock, is a major critical system problem. Widespread blood vessel dilation can cause vascular and volume shock and upper airway obstruction from swelling. Lower airway constriction results in wheezing and increased respiratory distress. The patient can die within a matter of minutes.

In the beginning, the patient may complain of itchy skin and hives with a scratchy or constricted feeling in the throat or swelling of the lips or tongue. The presence of symptoms above the neck is an ominous sign. Patients often report feeling a sense of impending doom. As the reaction becomes more severe, wheezing, stridor, facial swelling, nausea, vomiting, or diarrhea may develop. There will be weakness and mental status changes with the onset of shock. In the remote setting, early and aggressive treatment for anaphylaxis is warranted. Early treatment is especially important for the person with a history of severe anaphylaxis.

Treatment of Anaphylaxis: Specific ALS treatment with medication is required. Basic life support and PROP is appropriate but not definitive. In the backcountry we need to be concerned about both the immediate lifesaving treatment and long-term care. Appropriate wilderness medical treatment for anaphylaxis calls for the use of the medications epinephrine, diphenhydramine, and prednisone. These act to immediately reverse the effects of histamine and help prevent a recurrence of the problem over the next day or so. The recognition of severe anaphylaxis and the use of these medications is an important skill for the wilderness medical practitioner.

Anaphylaxis Treatment
WILDERNESS PROTOCOL

Epinephrine:

- 0.3 – 0.5 mg by intramuscular injection
- 1:1000 solution 1 mg = 1 ml
- Pediatric dose 0.15 mg (under 15 kg)
- Repeat as soon as 5 minutes if needed
- Action: reverses effects of histamine

Diphenhydramine:

- 25 - 50 mg by mouth
- Action: blocks histamine at receptor sites

Prednisone:

- 1 mg/kg up to 60 mg by mouth
- Action: anti-inflammatory, helps prevent biphasic reaction

Evacuation:

- Transport with additional epi on hand
- Not necessarily an emergency if treatment was successful

The drug epinephrine constricts blood vessels and dilates lower airway tubes, temporarily opposing the effects of histamine. This reduces swelling and respiratory distress and can reverse the onset of vascular and volume shock. It is best given by injection into the muscle of the lateral thigh at a dose of 0.3 milligram (mg). The patient's symptoms usually improve within ninety seconds. Repeat doses may be necessary if symptoms do not improve or begin to return after the first treatment.

Epinephrine is supplied specifically for the treatment of anaphylaxis in the form of a preloaded EpiPen or Twinject Autoinjector that automatically injects the right dose when pressed firmly against the skin. In the United States these devices are available only by prescription. Patients known to have severe allergies often carry one with them everywhere. In the backcountry setting it is advisable to carry two or three doses of epinephrine to cover reactions that recur while the antihistamine is taking effect. Practitioners trained and comfortable with syringes and ampoules may choose to carry epinephrine in that more economical and compact form.

The epinephrine injection is followed immediately by an oral dose of 50 mg of diphenhydramine, also known by its popular brand name Benadryl. This is an antihistamine that directly blocks the attachment of the histamine molecule to receptor sites on body tissues. Once it takes effect in fifteen to twenty minutes, repeat doses of epinephrine should no longer be necessary. Other antihistamines like loratadine or chlorpheniramine can also be effective as alternatives to diphenhydramine.

Diphenhydramine is available without a prescription in 25 mg tablets or capsules. A faster response may be obtained by using capsules and having the patient bite one open before swallowing. Warn the patient that the taste is very unpleasant.

Neither epinephrine nor diphenhydramine will remove the antigen or the histamine. It is possible to see symptoms return as the medication begins to wear off. Continued use of the antihistamine for a day or so may be necessary.

For offshore situations or long evacuations, adding the steroid drug prednisone at a dose of 40 to 60 mg once a day will suppress the inflammatory response mediated by histamine. This will further reduce the chance of the symptoms recurring. Prednisone can be used at this dose for up to five days. Like epinephrine, prednisone is a prescription drug; you will need authorization and instructions from your medical practitioner.

Because the effects of epinephrine are temporary, evacuation and medical follow-up should be planned. If the patient has recovered from the event, it need not be an emergency. Careful monitoring is crucial. ✚

Anaphylaxis
Wilderness Context

<u>High Risk Problem:</u>

- History of hospitalization for anaphylaxis
- Persistent abnormal mental status
- Incomplete response to treatment
- The patient is getting worse
- Second treatment needed

Chapter 8

Severe Asthma

Asthma is a chronic inflammatory disease causing lower airway constriction. The mechanism involves both spasm of the smooth muscle walls and swelling of the mucous membrane lining of the bronchial tubes. Acute asthma attacks are sometimes triggered by infection, cold air, exercise, or other stressors. Sometimes asthma flares without apparent reason. Some patients need to use medications daily to keep their asthma under control.

An acute asthma attack can be mild or severe. It can be a major critical system problem when it causes respiratory distress. If the initial spasm of smooth muscle is allowed to persist, the lower airway constriction will be exacerbated by secondary swelling.

Early signs and symptoms include respiratory distress, chest tightness, wheezing, and a dry cough. Most people with asthma are aware of the condition and familiar with the symptoms. They are usually relieved with self-administered medication such as inhaled albuterol that causes the smooth muscle to dilate.

Occasionally, an asthma attack will not respond to inhaled medication. This is usually due to the patient's waiting too long to administer it or other complications such as infection. Sometimes, the inhaler has been lost or has run out. Whatever the reason, when early treatment is delayed or ineffective, the initial spasm in the lower airways is made worse by secondary swelling. At this point, it will be difficult or impossible to deliver inhaled medication to the lower airways where it can exert its effect.

Asthma

Mechanism:
- Chronic inflammation of lower airways
- Acute exacerbations of bronchospasm and swelling
- Can be triggered by exercise, cold air, infection
- Can be mild or severe

Assessment:
- History of asthma
- Wheezing, coughing, chest tightness, respiratory distress

Severe respiratory distress can rapidly progress to respiratory failure. At this stage, respiration will be labored with the patient only able to speak one or two words between breaths. Emergency treatment is required. Like anaphylaxis, this can be a life-threatening problem that will not wait for evacuation or for medical help to be brought to the scene.

Treatment of Severe Asthma: You should first assist your patient in the proper use of his or her inhaler. Be sure that you are using the one with a fast-acting medication such as albuterol. The patient may recognize this as his or her "rescue inhaler." The distinction is important because some patients also use an inhaled steroid or other medication as an adjunct to therapy. These will not help in an acute attack.

Encourage the patient to inhale as deeply as possible while the inhaler is discharged into the mouth. The efficiency of the inhaler can be improved by the use of a spacer to contain the vapors while the patient inhales. This is simply a plastic tube with the inhaler on one end and the patient on the other. You can improvise a spacer by using a plastic water bottle with the bottom end cut off. Once the patient has inhaled the medication as deeply as possible, have him or her hold the medication in for a few seconds before exhaling.

It is safe to make several attempts to stop the asthma attack with an inhaler. However, do not delay moving to the next step if it is apparent that the patient cannot cooperate or is not improving. If use of the inhaler fails to reduce symptoms within a few minutes, the patient will need an injection of epinephrine.

Before inhaled drugs such as albuterol became available, epinephrine was a first-line treatment for an asthma attack. It is the same medication used for the emergency treatment of anaphylaxis. It is given in the same concentration and dose and by the same route. In this case we are taking advantage of the dilating effects that epinephrine has on the lower airways.

The dose of epinephrine is 0.3 mg injected into the thigh with an EpiPen or Twinject. The patient will usually feel better within a few minutes. One dose of epinephrine may completely abort the asthma attack, but a second dose may be given within as little as five minutes if needed. Once symptoms improve, the patient should self-administer his or her own MDI. If evacuation is impossible or prolonged, add a dose of prednisone given by mouth at 40 to 60 mg for an adult or 20 mg for a child. As with anaphylaxis, this will reduce lower airway inflammation and the chance of another attack during a long evacuation.

Anyone whose life you have just saved with epinephrine should be receiving follow-up medical care. If the symptoms are under control, this need not be an emergency. A safe, monitored evacuation is appropriate.

This emergency treatment is for use in severe respiratory distress caused by lower airway constriction in a known asthmatic. It is safe, effective, and carries little risk compared to the problems associated with prolonged respiratory distress. It is an important lifesaving skill for anyone responsible for asthmatic patients traveling in remote areas. ✚

Severe Asthma
Wilderness Context

<u>High-Risk Problem:</u>

- Persistent abnormal mental status.
- Incomplete response to treatment.
- MDI continues to be ineffective.
- The patient is getting worse.

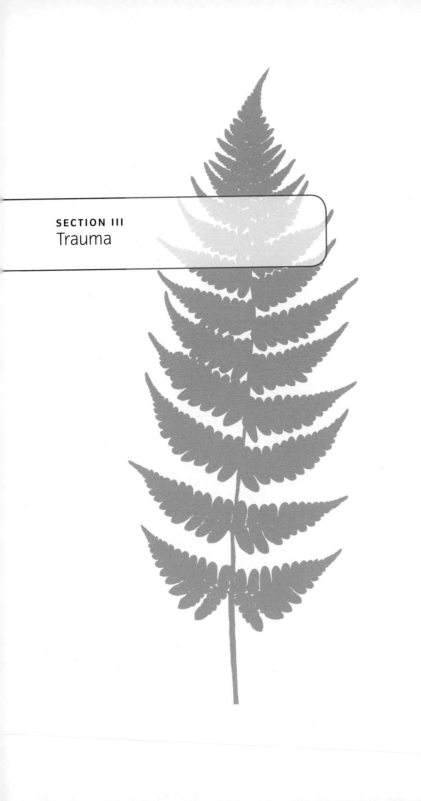

SECTION III
Trauma

Chapter 9
The Musculoskeletal System

After giving the X-rays one last look, I noted my final diagnosis on the chart: "Mildly displaced fracture of the distal radius." What this really means is "broken wrist" and the patient needs to see an orthopedic surgeon. Of course, she knew that when the accident happened three days ago.

Karen was rock climbing above Chimney Pond on the North Face of Katahdin when a toehold pulled loose, dropping her 6 feet onto a small ledge. Her partner, Steve, immediately took up the slack in the rope and looked up to see if Karen needed further help.

She had landed on her right wrist and felt a crack and immediate pain, but a minute or two passed while Karen checked her position and equipment before she was able to assess her own injuries. Her wrist hurt and felt swollen, and her fingers were tingling. She had no other apparent injuries, and her partner was able to lower her to the ground.

Steve conducted a patient survey and found that Karen was alert, fully oriented, and had no neck pain or tenderness. He noted the deformed and sore right wrist but continued his exam to be sure that it was the only injury. He used gentle traction to restore bone position, and a splint was fashioned using an aluminum stay from a backpack and a length of webbing for a sling. After a brief rest, the two climbers hiked back to the cabin.

As she warmed up, the return of normal color and sensation to Karen's fingers showed good blood perfusion beyond the injury. Even though she was pretty uncomfortable, and sometimes light-headed and nauseous for the next several hours, Karen knew that this was no emergency.

There was no mechanism of injury that could cause volume shock. Her feeling faint was part of a normal and harmless acute stress reaction. The splint effectively stabilized the wrist, and elevation and cold compresses controlled the swelling and pain. They continued to monitor the fingers to ensure circulation remained normal, and were able to safely wait out the storm that closed in for the next two days.

These two climbers recognized that this wrist injury was more of a logistical dilemma than a medical emergency, even though they knew it was fractured. Applying good common sense and basic understanding of the problem, they required neither rescue nor national news coverage.

Musculoskeletal injuries such as this are among the most common backcountry medical problems. Although they are often a major inconvenience, they are rarely emergencies. Contrast Karen's story with one of my other favorites: the rescue of a teenaged girl in the mountains of Wyoming. During the traverse of a scree slope, a falling rock crushed the end of one of her fingers. She was scared and

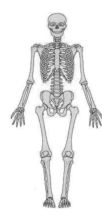

Musculoskeletal System

Structure:
bone, cartilage, tendon, ligament, muscle, fluid

Function:
support, mobility, protection

Problem:
stable injuries
unstable injuries
neurovascular injuries

in pain and became anxious, light-headed, and pale. Even though there was no mechanism for significant loss of blood volume, the trip leader decided that she was in shock and called for helicopter evacuation. The aircraft made an emergency flight in bad weather. Although it was very exciting and makes a great story, the risk to the helicopter and crew was totally unjustified. This patient was suffering only a crushed finger and acute stress reaction.

You already know that life- or limb-threatening emergency involves a major problem with the circulatory, respiratory, or nervous system. It is extremely important to recognize these problems when they occur. But in the backcountry it can be just as important to recognize when they don't.

If you've taken a first-aid course, you may recall a lot of concern over fractures of the thigh, skull, spine, pelvis, and ribs. It is important to realize here that the real problems are not the fractured bones themselves but the potential injury to the vital organs next to them. Trauma patients do not die of fractures, sprains, strains, and contusions. They die from airway obstruction, blood loss, and brain injury.

With a fractured femur or pelvis, we actually worry more about lacerated arteries, which are a major circulatory system problem. With fractured ribs we are concerned with the lungs, liver, or spleen. And with the skull or spine fractures, it is the brain and spinal cord inside that's of real importance. The first step in handling any musculoskeletal problem is ruling out a major injury to one of the critical body systems.

If your initial assessment discovers no existing critical system injury, you have given yourself the luxury of time: time to perform a secondary survey, think, treat, and safely evacuate yourself or your patient to medical care hours or days later. This may require help from a rescue team but rarely as a hurried or risky undertaking.

Structure and Function

Arms, legs, and fingers are moved by a system of cables, pulleys, and levers called tendons, ligaments, and bone. The motive power is supplied by the contraction of muscles working in balanced opposition across joints. The contraction of muscle on one side of the joint moves the bone one way; contraction on the other side moves it back.

Tendons are the tough connective tissue that join muscle to bone. Ligaments attach bone to bone across joints, and cartilage provides the smooth surfaces and padding where bones slide against each other. There are, of course, many types of bones and joints that make fascinating study. But knowing them in detail is not required for effective field treatment.

The spinal column with its stack of vertebrae is best viewed as another long bone with the head and pelvis as joints on either end. The same basic parts and principles are at work. The major difference is the complexity and importance of the adjacent soft tissue.

Musculoskeletal System Injury

The familiar medical terminology used to describe musculoskeletal injury includes contusion, strain, sprain, fracture, and dislocation. More terms are added to indicate position and relative severity of injuries, such as describing a sprain as "grade 1" for a minor tear in a ligament or "grade 3" for a complete rupture. Fractures can be comminuted, angulated, displaced, and described with a dozen other interesting terms. But for field treatment in the backcountry, the important distinction is simply whether the injury is stable or unstable. That is, can the injured part continue to perform its function without causing further injury, or does it need to be stabilized and referred to medical care?

Musculoskeletal Injury

Generic Assessment:
- Stable – can be used safely
- Unstable – must be stabilized and protected

Wilderness Context

Stable   Unstable

Because very few of us go into the backcountry with an X-ray machine, it is often impossible to tell if a bone is actually broken. In any case, ligament ruptures that don't show up on plain X-ray can be just as unstable. In the field, when an injury has the mechanism, signs, and symptoms of instability, we treat it as such. Most fractures, severe sprains, and all dislocations fall into this category.

Fractured bones and ruptured ligaments can result in unstable bone fragments and loose or displaced joints that can cause collateral damage to surrounding soft tissue. Of primary concern in extremity injury are the arteries, veins, and peripheral nerves that run adjacent to bones and joints. They tend to be grouped in a neurovascular bundle, much the way electrical wires and plumbing are fixed together as they run through a ship. These unprotected structures can be damaged during the initial injury or pinched by misalignment or swelling after the injury.

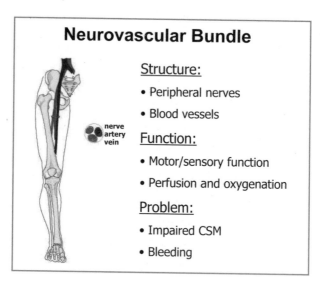

Neurovascular Bundle

nerve
artery
vein

Structure:
- Peripheral nerves
- Blood vessels

Function:
- Motor/sensory function
- Perfusion and oxygenation

Problem:
- Impaired CSM
- Bleeding

UNSTABLE EXTREMITY INJURY

Fractures, severe sprains and strains, and severe contusions in extremities can be caused by a variety of mechanisms reflecting the different ways force can be applied to bones and joints. The injury may be caused by leverage, twisting, direct impact, or a piece of bone being pulled away where the tendon or ligament attaches to it. For field purposes defining mechanism of injury can be generalized to a yes or no question: Was there sufficient force to cause a fracture or rupture a ligament?

I know what's coming next: "So what's sufficient force?" You're going to tell me about your Aunt Mable who broke her hip just stepping off a curb. You'll mention your friend who limped around on stress fractures for weeks before being diagnosed, and he didn't fall or anything. I agree with you; sufficient force can be difficult to define.

It is easy to recognize a positive mechanism of injury with the long falls and high-speed impacts typical of climbing or skiing accidents. The cases that obviously lack mechanism, like waking up with a sore neck after sleeping on a rock ledge, are also easy. It's the ones in between that really need a careful scene survey and history.

To the vague definition of "sufficient force" we add the not-so-vague signs and symptoms of instability. Combined with mechanism of injury, these provide a fairly clear guideline for identifying injuries that are likely to involve broken bones or other unstable elements such as severe sprains.

Signs and Symptoms of Unstable Injury

- The inability to move, use, or bear weight within a short time after injury.
- The rapid onset of pain, tenderness, and swelling.
- A history of feeling or hearing a "snap, crack, or pop."
- Obvious deformity or angulation.
- The sensation of grating of bones against each other (crepitus) on movement.
- The patient or examiner feels instability of bones or joints.
- Impaired CSM.

Unstable Injury

Signs and Symptoms:

- Instability – sign or symptom
- Crepitus – sign or symptom
- Inability to use, move, or bear weight
- Deformity or angulation
- Impaired CSM

"Combined with mechanism of injury, these provide a fairly clear guideline for identifying injuries that are likely to involve…unstable elements…"

For example, consider two nearly identical swollen and sore knees on two nearly identically disgruntled skiers. Patient number one fell skiing early in the morning, twisting the knee. After resting for a few minutes, he was able to continue skiing well into the afternoon with only minor discomfort. The knee became sore and stiff after he stopped skiing for the day and soaked in a hot tub. It is now late evening and his knee is quite swollen and he can barely move it.

Patient number two fell only sixty minutes ago, feeling a sharp pop and immediate pain. After the pain decreased a bit, he tried to continue down the mountain but the knee "gave out," leaving him unable to control his skis. He presented to the clinic in a ski patrol toboggan and is now quite swollen and immobile.

Both of these patients are grumpy and uncomfortable, and the pain prohibits a reliable examination of the knee. It is the history that makes the difference in assessment. The first skier's story does not fit the description of an unstable injury. He was able to continue using his knee for a while after the accident without any sense of instability. His severe discomfort twelve hours later is the result of the swelling and pressure in the joint that typically develops slowly after minor injury. The hot tub didn't help any either.

Patient number two, with the sharp pop and the knee that gives out on him, clearly has an unstable injury. It is probably a ligament rupture and may or may not include a fracture. If he were to continue to ski, he could have caused damage to the neurovascular bundle running behind the knee. Appropriate field treatment required stabilization and evacuation to medical care. His pain is due primarily to the rapid swelling from bleeding inside the joint.

Treatment of Unstable Extremity Injury: An extremity fracture or sprain by itself is never an emergency, but we need to protect the neurovascular bundle and other soft tissue from further damage. The most important anticipated problem is extremity ischemia caused by lacerated or kinked blood vessels. Perfusion can also be lost when splints or bandages are tied too tightly. Treating the fracture or sprain correctly will fix or prevent these problems.

As we've said, nervous system tissue is the most sensitive to oxygen deprivation. With the onset of ischemia, peripheral nerves stop functioning and the extremity goes numb. With continued ischemia the control of movement is lost as well. The inevitable result of prolonged ischemia is infarction of tissue. This makes the ongoing assessment of the neurovascular bundle one of your primary concerns during long-term care.

The method of assessment for nerve function is checking circulation, sensation, and movement (abbreviated CSM). You have experienced problems with CSM if you've slept on your arm or kept your backpack straps too tight. Circulation is impaired, your arm goes numb, and then you can't move it. As circulation is restored, movement returns, then tingling, then full sensation.

Circulation is checked by looking for evidence of blood flow in the injured extremity. Can you detect any pulses beyond ("distal" to) an area of injury? Is the skin normal in color, or pale or blue? Is the skin colder than the same extremity on the other side?

It is not unusual for an extremity to feel numb or cold immediately following injury, especially if the injury results in deformity or the patient is having an acute stress reaction. Your treatment will usually result in a significant improvement in

CSM status as circulation is restored. CSM may decay later as swelling develops under a splint or wrap. You will need to keep watching it.

Extremity tissue can usually survive up to two hours of ischemia with minimal damage. Beyond this, the risk of tissue death and permanent damage increases quickly with time. If your treatment efforts do not succeed in restoring CSM, you have a limb-threatening emergency. Immediate evacuation is indicated if conditions permit.

The generic treatment for unstable extremity injury has three distinct phases: traction into position, hand stable, and splint stable.

Unstable Injury
Long Bones

Treatment:

1. Traction Into Position
2. Hand Stable
3. Splint Stable
4. Check CSM before and after

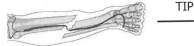

TIP

"Your patient will be reassured to hear that traction into position is intended to be a slow and gentle process."

Traction into Position: Injured bones and joints, and the soft tissues around them, are much more comfortable and much less likely to be damaged further if splinted in normal anatomic position. While many injured extremities will remain in good position or return there on their own, some will require help from you.

To restore anatomic position of a displaced bone we first apply traction. This separates bone ends and reduces pain. Then, while traction is maintained, normal position is restored. To understand how this works, picture moving a chain as a unit by holding the links under tension, rather than allowing them to rattle against each other.

Shaft fractures of long bones are brought into the line of normal bone axis, the "in line" position. This is where the effect of opposing muscles is most balanced and the blood circulation to the extremity beyond the injury is best maintained. If you're not sure what the realigned extremity should look like, check the other side. That's why people have two of almost everything.

Injured joints, such as elbows, shoulders, and knees, usually do not need to be repositioned. If your patient is conscious and mobile, he will have already found the most comfortable position for the injured joint and be holding it there by the time you come along. If the patient is unable to move the injured joint, splinting in the position found is best unless distal CSM is impaired.

In severely deformed joints with CSM impairment, TIP with movement toward the mid-range position is used until circulation is reestablished. In some specific cases, which we'll discuss later, TIP can be used to reduce the dislocation, putting the dislocated joint back in normal position. This almost always fixes any problems with distal CSM.

TIP is a safe procedure if done properly. It generally decreases pain rather than increases it. However, to be successful it helps to have the cooperation and confidence of the injured person. Pulling on a fractured leg without telling its owner how or why you're going to do it won't win you any friends. If necessary, you and your assistants may want to practice on an uninjured limb first.

Occasionally it will be impossible to comfortably and safely restore position, even using TIP. You should discontinue TIP and stabilize the injury in the position found if TIP causes a significant increase in pain or if movement of the extremity is prevented by resistance.

Open fractures with bone ends protruding through the skin are still managed with TIP. Bone ends are often pulled beneath the skin surface when traction is applied, so it is best to first clean the exposed bone by irrigating with water and brushing away debris. Clean the surrounding skin with antiseptic solution or soap and water. Try to keep the skin of the wound edges from becoming trapped under the bone as you realign the fracture. You may have to pull it free with a clean tweezers or gloved finger as the bone is manipulated back into the wound.

Hand Stable: Once you have repositioned an extremity injury, stability must be maintained until the splint can take over. This may mean having someone hold gentle traction on the extremity while you collect materials. If you don't have an army of assistants, you may have to use snow, rocks, or pieces of equipment to hold the limb in place. Don't just drop it without some kind of support. Of course, if you were really thinking, you might have had your splint materials ready *before* you started the process.

Splint Stable: Splinting is a real art in first aid. We've seen an incredible variety of splints from the fabulously expensive stainless steel jobs with dozens of moving parts, to the disorganized collections of fire wood and bailing twine. The best of them are simple, light, cheap, and probably in your backpack or boat right now. The most useful splinting materials include sleeping pads, backpack stays, snowshoes, flotation vests, nylon webbing, and giant safety pins.

What . . . you don't carry giant safety pins? You should. This marvelous device (aka a diaper pin) weighs practically nothing, takes up no space, and costs only a few cents, yet can convert a shirt or jacket into an instant sling and swathe for wrist, arm, and shoulder injuries. It is almost as useful as duct tape, the other item you should never leave home without.

Duct tape is that silver stuff that is very sticky and strong, yet easy to tear into pieces with your hands. It can be warmed with a lighter in cold and wet weather and will stick to almost any surface. With a few yards of duct tape and that giant safety pin, you can splint or fix just about everything. In addition, there is one commercial splint material worthy of mention. It is called a SAM Splint™ and consists of a strip of malleable aluminum sandwiched between layers of foam padding. It can be bent and cut to create a variety of lightweight but strong splints for the wrist, ankle, and fingers.

Splint Stable

Complete:
- Provides stability and protection

Comfortable:
- No pressure points or abrasion
- Can be adjusted

Compact:
- Only as large as necessary
- Allows for CSM checks

Principles of Splinting: Regardless of how you make it, an improvised splint should be *complete, comfortable,* and *compact*. Be sure to pay attention to all three qualities. Duct taping someone's arm to a canoe would do a fine job of immobilizing their wrist but wouldn't be very comfortable. The evacuation would be dangerous, to say the least. Splints should be:

Complete—Splint in normal anatomic position, if possible, including the joint above and below the injury. For example: To effectively splint a lower leg fracture, the ankle and knee must be immobilized. Splints for joint injuries include the bones above and below the injury. For example: To splint the elbow, the forearm and upper arm are included in the splint. There is no need to include adjacent joints in the splint. The shoulder and wrist may be left mobile.

Comfortable—Splints should be well padded, strong, and snug. There should be no movement of the injured bones, or any pressure points or loose spots. Your splint should improve and preserve blood perfusion and nerve function, not impair it. A good splint results in decreased pain and intact CSM.

Compact—A splint should be no larger or more complex than necessary. It should allow you to monitor distal CSM, and loosen or adjust the splint if ischemia develops. It should not inhibit the evacuation that you have in mind.

Once the extremity is stabilized with your perfect splint, and you are satisfied that CSM is improving, treatment should include rest and elevation to reduce swelling and pressure. As long as distal CSM remains normal or continues to improve, you can take your time planning a safe and comfortable evacuation.

Joint Dislocations

Joint Structure:
bone, cartilage, tendon, muscle, ligament, fluid

Function:
support, mobility

Problem:
disability
pain
ischemia

JOINT DISLOCATIONS

The average garden variety joint is a complex, mobile assembly of bones, ligaments, cartilage, tendon, and muscle. To the delight of orthopedic surgeons everywhere, these structures can be injured in a wide variety of combinations and levels of severity. A dislocation occurs when enough force is applied to the bone to tear the restraining ligaments and allow the joint to come apart.

By definition, dislocations have the mechanism of injury, signs, and symptoms of unstable injuries, and we treat them by the same general principals: stabilize the joint in the position found and evacuate to treatment. There are, however, three specific dislocations that deserve special attention because they are easy and safe to reduce in the field. These are simple dislocations of the shoulder, patella (knee-cap), and digits (fingers and toes). This can save a lot of pain and trouble and make you into a real hero by transforming a gruesome medical emergency into a minor logistical problem.

Joint Dislocations
WILDERNESS PROTOCOL

Treatment:

Immediate field reduction if:

- Simple dislocation from indirect force
- Shoulder, patella, digits
- Wilderness context
- Patient consents

"The damage to the joint and surrounding soft tissue due to ischemia will increase significantly after a couple of hours."

SHOULDER DISLOCATIONS

Simple dislocations are caused by indirect injury, where force is applied at a distance from the joint and the dislocation is caused by leverage or torque. The usual mechanism is forced external rotation and abduction. This movement is similar to raising your arm to throw a baseball, high bracing with a kayak paddle, or catching a fall on an outstretched arm while skiing. Fractures are uncommon and generally do not interfere with treatment.

These injuries can be extremely uncomfortable and result in significant ischemia to the joint and surrounding soft tissue. Damage will increase significantly after a couple of hours. The benefit of early field reduction, even by an inexperienced rescuer, generally outweighs the risk of causing further damage with manipulation. Reduction is best accomplished within an hour of the injury, before severe swelling and muscle spasm develops.

The more serious dislocation from direct injury is usually the result of a high-speed impact into a solid object. Distinguishing this mechanism from that of indirect force is usually not too difficult. These injuries are almost always associated with other major trauma.

You will be trying to identify those simple dislocations caused by indirect force that may be fixed in the field. This is where careful attention to the mechanism of injury during your surveys and history can really pay off. The patient will describe the classic mechanism, frequently with a history of recurrent dislocation in the same extremity. You'll notice right away that the person with a dislocated shoulder is in moderate to severe discomfort. Acute stress reaction is common. In about half of the cases there is some CSM impairment of the arm and hand. The shoulder itself loses the rounded contour and becomes a "step off" deformity with a hollow area where the shoulder is normally full and rounded. The patient will be unwilling to move the shoulder joint at all without help and coaching.

Occasionally, a shoulder dislocation can be confused with a shoulder *separation*. A separation refers to disruption of the joint between the distal end of the clavicle and the scapula. This is called the acromioclavicular joint, or AC joint. The usual mechanism of injury is a direct blow to the top of the shoulder during a fall. This joint lies directly above the shoulder joint and can produce a lump that can be mistaken for the "step off" deformity. However, the shoulder joint and upper arm will remain mobile. In a shoulder dislocation mobility is lost.

Treatment of Shoulder Dislocation: The simple dislocation of the shoulder should be reduced in the field if the evacuation time to definitive care will be greater than two hours. It should also be considered if the evacuation will be exceptionally difficult or dangerous to perform while the shoulder remains displaced. These criteria apply to most backcountry and marine situations.

There are a number of techniques that are effective in reducing dislocated shoulders. The best we've found for field use requires only a small patch of level ground and one rescuer. Because it is performed gently and slowly, it carries a low risk of causing further injury.

To begin, the patient's arm is supported while being moved to a position lying on his back. Gentle traction on the upper arm will help relieve pain during movement. The patient's cooperation and relaxation is essential. This will take some time. There is no reason to torture your patient with speed. Once the patient is lying on his back, the rescuer applies gentle traction to the arm and slowly swings it into a position about 90 degrees from the body with the elbow bent.

The rescuer continues to hold gentle TIP with one hand just above the elbow. With the other hand on the patient's forearm, the rescuer gently and slowly externally rotates the arm until the "baseball position" is reached. This looks just like it sounds. It is exactly the position the patient would have his arm if he were throwing a ball. Once the arm is in position, make *yourself* comfortable.

Now, traction should become firm but not enough to slide the patient across the ground. There should be no need for countertraction unless you are working on a slipper surface like ice or snow. The patient should be gently and repeatedly encouraged to relax his shoulder muscles. Tell him that he must let the joint return to its normal position with the muscles in balance.

Usually within five to ten minutes, and often a lot sooner, the muscles will fatigue, allowing the joint to slip back into place. If nothing has happened after about fifteen minutes, try a move called "throwing the baseball." Again, this is exactly like sounds.

Watch the patient's shoulder and pick a moment when you see the muscles really relax. Gently rotate the arm and hand forward as if the patient were throwing a ball. This is almost always successful in encouraging the shoulder to pop back into its socket.

Shoulder Reduction

Baseball Position:

• Slowly abduct and rotate the arm away from the body.

Usually best if the patient lays on the ground or deck.

• Apply steady, firm traction while encouraging the patient to relax the shoulder muscles.

• Reduction may take up to 15 minutes.

You will know when the shoulder joint has been reduced by the dramatic relief of pain and return of mobility of the joint. You can often feel and see a sudden shift of the upper arm as it relocates in the socket. If CSM impairment was present before reduction, it will rapidly improve afterward. Remember to check and document CSM both before and after reduction.

Following reduction, your patient usually experiences significant relief and will thank you profusely enough to become embarrassing. Enjoy it, but remember that a joint dislocation has the positive mechanism, signs, and symptoms of an unstable injury. Inevitably, swelling and pressure will develop and pain will increase over time. The most effective splint is a simple sling. The patient should plan for medical follow-up within a week, if possible.

Some shoulders will remain quite painful immediately after reduction. This is especially true of dislocations in which a small piece of bone is chipped off the ball of the upper arm. As long as distal CSM is intact, this should not be a cause for alarm. You're treating for unstable injury anyway, but early medical follow-up is a good idea.

Dislocations that result from direct force are generally more complicated and usually not reduced in the field. Manipulation is directed only at restoring CSM if necessary and positioning the patient for safe evacuation. If the patient is to be walked out, a sling pinned to the patient's shirt or jacket is effective immobilization.

Shoulder – Post Reduction

Long-Term Care:

- Monitor distal CSM. Ischemia is an anticipated problem.

- Ice, NSAIDs. Swelling and pain are anticipated problems.

- Sling, limit ROM to avoid abduction and external rotation.

- Evacuation to medical care, non-emergent if CSM is OK and pain is tolerable.

PATELLA DISLOCATION

The patella, better known as the kneecap, is an isolated bone embedded as a kind of fulcrum in the quadriceps tendon. This large tendon transmits the powerful force of the quadriceps muscle in the front of the thigh to the front of the lower leg to allow you to extend the knee. This is the motion you'd use to bring your foot forward, kick a ball, or kick your climbing partner for dropping you.

The quadriceps tendon passes over and through a groove in the femur, like a cable through a pulley. In patellar dislocation the cable slips off the femur, making it impossible for the knee to function.

Like the shoulder, the patella can dislocate with a direct blow or an indirect mechanism, typically a sudden extension of the knee while twisting or turning. The patient often has a history of recurrent dislocation. A dislocation from indirect mechanism is always lateral, leaving the patella pinned against the outside of the knee by the pull of the quadriceps.

The appearance can be deceiving. Shifting the patella laterally will make the bony prominence on the inside of the knee stand out and look like the missing patella. Don't be fooled. Feel for the patella laterally—you'll find it.

Like the shoulder, these dislocations also are extremely uncomfortable, and there is little or no motion of the joint possible. Distal circulation and sensation is usually unaffected, but you should check it anyway. Damage to surrounding soft tissue will increase with time, as will the difficulty of reduction.

Treatment of Patella Dislocation: Like the shoulder, a dislocated patella should be reduced if the evacuation time will be greater than two hours or the evacuation will be unreasonably difficult. Reducing a dislocated patella is also reversing the mechanism of injury. Take the tension off the tendon by flexing the hip, and then straighten the knee. If the patella does not relocate on its own, a gentle push with your thumbs will usually do the trick. Like the shoulder, relief of pain and return of mobility will indicate success. Also like the shoulder, these injuries are likely to result in swelling and significant pain later.

Ideally, a reduced patella dislocation should be splinted as an unstable injury and carried out. In less than ideal situations, the knee could be braced and the patient walked out if pain permits. The key is to avoid repeating the mechanism of injury. As long as distal CSM is okay, there is no emergency, but medical follow-up is important.

Patella Post Reduction

Long-Term Care:

- Ice, NSAIDs. Swelling and pain are anticipated problems.

- Splint or tape to limit ROM and keep patella in mid-line.

- Carry-out evacuation is ideal, but walk-out is OK if patella is stabilized.

"As long as CSM is OK, there is no emergency, but medical follow-up is important."

DIGIT DISLOCATIONS

Joints in the fingers and toes usually dislocate due to an indirect force that levers the bone ends apart. The classic example is catching a falling softball the wrong way. Other examples include catching a disappearing canoe wrong, catching a falling climber wrong, or just having your hand in the wrong place at the wrong time. In any case, what you end up with is a finger pointing the wrong way at the distal or middle joint.

These dislocations are often an associated small chip fracture. Motion of the dislocated joint is impossible, and there will be some degree of CSM impairment. Like all dislocations, damage from ischemia will increase with time.

Treatment of Digit Dislocation: Your first reaction when confronted with a dislocated finger or toe will be to want it back where it belongs, especially if it is yours. Fortunately this is exactly what should be done if definitive care will be delayed more than two hours. TIP is the same as for shaft fractures; pull in the normal axis of the digit. Reduction will be most easily accomplished right after the injury has occurred and before the swelling and pain get worse.

After getting your patient's consent, simply grasp the end of the offending finger with one hand and the rest of the finger in the other. Slowly but firmly pull the end of the finger first in the direction it is pointing and, while maintaining traction, swing it back in line. This is not as easy as it sounds, but it does work. You'll probably need to wrap the end of your patient's finger in gauze or a bandanna to help keep your grip.

You can confirm a successful reduction by checking range of motion, but resist the temptation to play with it. Remember, fracture is very likely and it will need medical attention at some point. So splint it in the mid-range of the joint's motion and give it a rest. A simple and elegant way to do this is to buddy tape the finger to the adjacent healthy digit. Put a gauze pad or piece of cloth between the fingers first. Again, don't forget to check CSM before and after reduction. Things should improve with your treatment.

Digit Dislocation

Reduction:

- TIP to normal anatomy
- Check ROM and distal CSM

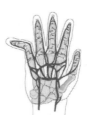

Long-Term care:

- Pain-free activity only
- Anticipate pain and swelling
- Splint or buddy tape to next digit
- Medical follow-up, non-emergent if CSM is OK

Difficult Dislocations: In the backcountry any dislocation that resists your efforts at reduction can become a serious problem. Pain may be severe, and the potential for tissue damage due to ischemia increases with time. If CSM is significantly impaired and cannot be restored by traction and repositioning, immediate evacuation to medical care is warranted. These are limb-threatening emergencies.

Spine, Femur, and Pelvis Injuries

In stabilizing musculoskeletal injuries to the spine, pelvis, and femur, we apply the same assessment skills and splinting principles as in extremity injury. Effective splinting of these bones usually requires a long backboard, vacuum splint, or litter that can secure the hips, back, and neck. Needless to say, this pretty well eliminates walking your patient out of the woods in all but the most desperate situations.

The equipment necessary is brought to the scene by rescue teams or aircraft and requires a carry-out or airlift evacuation. While you are waiting, you will need to shelter and stabilize the patient in place, or move her to shelter in a safe location.

SPINE INJURY

The possibility of spine injury has long been a major concern for emergency medical personnel. The delicate tissue of the spinal cord, really an extension of the brain, is surrounded and protected by the bones, ligaments, cartilage, and muscles that make up the spinal column. The worry is that an unstable spinal column injury could cause or exacerbate injury to the spinal cord during extrication and transport. This is similar to the concern over an unstable extremity injury causing or exacerbating an injury to the adjacent neurovascular bundle, except that the consequences can be more severe.

The neck is the most commonly injured area because it is the most mobile section of the spine, linking the heavy mass of the head with the body. As a result it is prone to injury, which snaps the head back and forth like a ball on a string. It is also subject to damage when a force is applied to the top of the head, such as being struck by a rock fall or diving into shallow water. There is a logical association between head and neck injury.

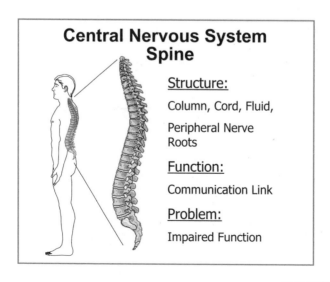

Central Nervous System Spine

Structure:

Column, Cord, Fluid,

Peripheral Nerve Roots

Function:

Communication Link

Problem:

Impaired Function

Injury to the thoracic spine (chest level) is much less common due to the added rigidity of the rib cage. This is the most stable area of the spine, and injury at this level is more likely to be associated with other major chest trauma from significant force.

Below the thorax is the lumbar spine, which, like the neck, is less protected and more mobile. Unstable injuries are more common here but cord injury is rare. Near the top of the lumbar spine, the cord separates into individual nerve roots that look like a loose bundle of linguine. These nerve roots are much more mobile and less likely to be injured by pressure or impact.

The signs and symptoms of unstable spine injury are really no different from those involved in other musculoskeletal trauma. But because the consequences of spinal cord injury can be so devastating, we tend to be much more conservative in our assessment and treatment. Persistent pain and tenderness, the inability to move easily, deformity, or crepitis should alert you to the possibility of an unstable spinal column injury.

Any neurologic impairment, such as numbness, tingling or muscle weakness, suggests the possibility of spinal cord involvement. This has far more serious implications than the injury to the bones and ligaments, just like impaired distal CSM in an extremity injury. Any spine injury with persistent CSM impairment should be considered an emergency. The ideal treatment is stabilization and urgent evacuation to neurosurgical care.

Spinal column injury without evidence of spinal cord involvement in an awake and oriented patient can be treated like other musculoskeletal problems. Signs and symptoms of unstable injury require splinting, protection, and evacuation to medical care. In the absence of other serious problems, this need not be an emergency.

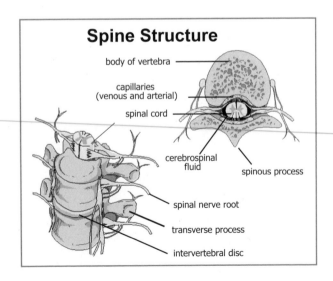

Spine Structure

body of vertebra

capillaries
(venous and arterial)

spinal cord

cerebrospinal
fluid

spinous process

spinal nerve root

transverse process

intervertebral disc

If your patient's mental status is altered due to brain injury, intoxication, or ASR, your assessment will be unreliable. In this case, a significant mechanism for spine injury should motivate you to stabilize the spine no matter what your exam shows or the patient tells you. You can evaluate again later when your patient may have cleared her head, calmed down, or sobered up.

Treatment of Spine Injury: For field purposes the spine is treated as a long bone with a joint at each end. The positioning and treatment principles are the same although we don't use traction. Gentle realignment is used to restore the injured spine to the normal anatomic position with the head level with the shoulders and pelvis and the eyes forward. As with other long bones, normal anatomic position will be most stable and least likely to injure adjacent nerves and blood vessels.

Hand stable for the spine involves maintaining normal alignment throughout any lifting, rolling, or carrying. The next step is splint stable with the head and neck secured with a collar, and the rest of the splint completed with a long board or litter, which stabilizes the lower spine and pelvis. Splinting is best accomplished with equipment designed for this purpose.

Spine Injury Treatment

Field Treatment:

- Restore spine alignment
- Package for protection and stability
- Treat pain, monitor for change
- Evacuate; urgent if...
  - persistent neurological deficit
  - palpable deformity
  - other critical system injury
  - severe pain

A comfortable and effective cervical collar can be improvised from jacket, sleeping bag, or tarp wrapped around the neck from behind and crossed under the chin. This will help reduce neck motion while avoiding the pressure and abrasion problems associated with rigid extrication collars in the long-term-care setting. Whole body stabilization with an improvised litter is possible, but a litter manufactured for this purpose is going to be a lot easier to handle.

In most cases you will be better off setting up camp right where you are and sending a runner for help. While you're waiting, lay your patient on a pad and sleeping bag for comfort and insulation. You can "block" the head with packs or clothing to prevent excessive movement. She will need help with everything, including eating, drinking, urinating, and defecating. Because your patient will be unable to exercise to generate body heat, you must be careful to keep her well fed and hydrated, warm, and dry.

If waiting for rescue is not an option, you should provide the maximum stability possible to the spine before movement. Carrying the patient supine in an improvised litter with a cervical collar in place is best. There are times, however, when the benefits of stabilizing the patient are outweighed by the risks presented by an unstable scene or high-risk evacuation. Having a person walk or climb in spite of a possible unstable spine injury should be viewed as a last resort, but occasionally necessary in the real world. When you have no choice but to move immediately, you can take some comfort in the knowledge that unstable spine injury is very rare and the probability of further injury is remote. Try to maintain alignment during rapid extrication, if possible, and complete your stabilization as soon as the risk is minimized.

Remember, we are modifying the plan, not the diagnosis. The reasons should appear in your problem list. You might note that problem number one is an unstable spine injury. Problem number two might be the fact that the wind has shifted and your hotshot crew is about to be overrun by a wildfire.

Spine Stabilization
Wilderness Context

<u>High-Risk Environment:</u>
- Rapid extrication, then clear or stabilize
- Stabilize in recovery position
- Allow sitting, standing, or walking
- Soft or partial stabilization
- Modify the plan, not the diagnosis!

"Examples include patients or rescuers threatened by a wild-land fire, avalanche, or hypothermia."

FEMUR FRACTURES

The femur is part of the lower extremity and structurally is similar to the other long bones in the leg and arm, but much bigger. It is not easy to fracture a femur. Massive force is required.

We group femur fracture with spine and pelvis injuries because, unlike the other extremities, they require whole body stabilization. The hip and pelvis form the joint above the injury, requiring a litter or backboard to secure. The powerful thigh muscles are easily thrown into spasm by movement.

Of the signs and symptoms of fracture, the one most typical of the femur is severe pain. Unless there is pain masking from other injury or intoxication, these patients will be very uncomfortable. They do not smile, laugh, or ask questions. They hurt. Movement is difficult, and weight bearing is impossible.

A femur fracture should make you think of volume shock. The large femoral artery runs close to the bone and can be lacerated by broken bone ends. Even in a closed fracture of the femur, considerable blood can be lost into the thigh. The *original* problem may be a fractured femur, but the more serious *anticipated problem* is volume shock.

Treatment of Femur Fracture: Traction into position will help reduce spasm and the chance of injury to arteries and nerves. It also may reduce pain, but this is not always the case. Traction should be maintained until splinting is completed.

The ideal femur splint for backcountry use is a well-padded litter or vacuum mattress. Specialized traction splints may also be used by trained rescuers but tend to cause skin ischemia and are difficult to package for carry-out or helicopter evacuation. Improvised traction splints employing ski poles, canoe paddles, and other pieces of equipment are often more architecturally interesting than medically useful.

A femur fracture should be considered an emergency, more so if there is any evidence of distal CSM impairment or volume shock. In spite of the fact that your patient will be going into surgery at some point, you must continue to feed and hydrate him to avoid dehydration and hypothermia. Either condition will complicate his already significant problems.

Femur Fracture
Wilderness Context

- High-Risk Problem: A' is shock and impaired CSM

- Stabilize in vacuum mattress or litter

- NPO if evac is short and hypothermia/dehydration is not an issue

- ALS intercept for pain control and fluid

- No traction splint for long evacuation

PELVIC FRACTURES

Like the femur, it takes a significant force to fracture the pelvis. These are usually the injuries of long falls, high-speed ski accidents, and avalanches. Like the femur, a major concern is the possibility of severe bleeding from arteries and veins adjacent to the fracture site. Volume shock should be on your anticipated problem list if it's not already present.

Pelvic fractures are a little tricky. They are usually quite painful, but not always. They can also be difficult to distinguish from hip or lower lumbar spine fractures. There are no single outstanding signs or symptoms. In the presence of positive mechanism, pelvic pain and tenderness, and inability to bear weight, you have little choice but to treat for fracture.

Treatment of Pelvic Fractures: Because of danger to adjacent blood vessels, possible pelvic fractures deserve litter stabilization also. Unless the spine is involved, it is not necessary to use a cervical collar. If the pelvis is clearly unstable, a pelvic binding may help reduce the movement of bone fragments while reducing the space available for internal blood loss. This can be as simple as a tarp wrapped broadly around the pelvis at the level of the hips, pulled tight, and tied. A padded hip belt from a backpack will also work. As with the femur, it is often going to be best to stabilize in place and call for help with evacuation.

Pelvic Fracture
Wilderness Context

- High Risk Problem: A' is shock and impaired CSM

- Stabilize in vacuum mattress or litter

- NPO if evacuation is short and hypothermia and dehydration is not an issue

- ALS intercept for pain control and fluid

- Pelvic binding may reduce internal bleeding

STABLE INJURIES

Nearly every morning, even before the lifts have opened, there are a couple of skiers waiting for the clinic to open. Anyone in ski area medicine will recognize them: one leg stiff, furrowed brow, frown on the face. This is the stable knee injury.

Paul had been skiing the snowfields above King Pine chair yesterday when he caught a ski tip on a tree, twisting the lower leg outward. He felt mild pain in the right knee but was able to continue skiing for several more hours.

He felt no pop or snap at the time of injury and no instability afterward. It was not until later in the evening that the pain and swelling began. He soaked in the hot tub for an hour and went to bed. Remember this guy?

Today Paul's knee is very sore. There is slight swelling and tenderness on the inside of the joint. There is good range of motion but with considerable pain. Even with these findings today, however, the history indicates that Paul has a stable injury.

The treatment for Paul's injury is Rest, Ice, Compression, and Elevation, abbreviated **RICE.** During the first forty-eight hours after injury, heat should not be applied because it will just increase the swelling. After a day or so, Paul can begin pain-free activity, that is, whatever activity he can do without causing an increase in pain. He should be ready to ski again in a few days or weeks.

The typical signs and symptoms of stable injury include positive mechanism and pain but none of the specific signs and symptoms of instability. The patient is able to use, move, or bear weight within the first hour following injury. There is no history of a "snap, crack, or pop." There is no deformity, crepitus, or sense of instability.

Swelling is common but develops slowly over several hours from the accumulation of edema fluid rather than rapidly from bleeding. It is not unusual for the patient to experience considerable pain and immobility the next day as this swelling and pressure reaches its peak. This is especially true if he continued to use the injured part for a while after the injury or indulged in a hot tub.

Stable Injuries

S/sx:

- No deformity, no instability on exam
- No sense of instability reported by patient
- Able to move and bear weight after accident
- Distal CSM intact
- Slow onset of swelling
- Pain proportional to apparent injury

Treatment of Stable Injuries: The ideal early treatment of stable injuries is essentially the same as unstable. This conservative treatment prevents the development of disability from excessive pain and swelling during the first twenty-four hours. The handy mnemonic is **RICE:**

R–Rest; local rest = splinted or limited use
I–Ice; use as tolerated first twenty-four hours.
C–Compression; i.e., ACE bandage. Use only on distal extremity.
E–Elevation; raise the injury above heart level

Pain-Free Activity (PFA): After the first twenty-four hours, or when most of the pain and swelling has resolved, the injured person may perform whatever activity is possible as long as additional pain is not caused. This may include skiing, or it may require very limited use around camp for several days.

Medication: Anti-inflammatory medication such as aspirin or ibuprofen can help reduce swelling and discomfort. Using the medication regularly for several days works better than taking it occasionally in response to pain.

Elevation and rest are the most important elements of RICE and most useful early on while the swelling is likely to be the worst. Ice is also very helpful. Even in the summer, you can achieve some cooling by evaporation by wrapping the injury in a water-soaked bandage.

Following these treatment guidelines, all stable injuries should show steady improvement. If not, your patient is being too active, or your assessment may be wrong. It *is* possible to have a stable injury with a small fracture causing prolonged discomfort. Never be afraid to reassess the situation and change your mind. Medical people do it all the time.

Stable Injuries

Treatment:

- Rest, ice, compression, elevation
- Pain-free activity
- Splint or sling for comfort
- NSAIDs for pain and swelling
- Monitor CSM
- Medical follow-up when possible

Tendinitis

This is a good time to talk about the meaning of the suffix "itis." It is a nonspecific term indicating inflammation or irritation. Tendinitis is inflammation of a tendon, arthritis is inflammation of a joint, appendicitis is inflammation of the appendix. It does not specify *why* the part is inflamed. The cause may be infection, trauma, sunburn . . . anything capable of causing damage. "Itis" is really a symptom of a more specific problem.

In the case of tendons, muscles, ligaments, and cartilage, the usual cause in wilderness travel is overuse, or "repetitive motion injury." Anything subject to repeated friction will wear out eventually; ropes, sails, boot soles, your favorite toothbrush. Your body parts are no exception. What is exceptional about your body is its ability to repair the damage if you can give it enough time.

Tendinitis, like the kind that develops in a kayaker's wrist, is a symptom of too much wear and too little time for repair. You will note the typical pain, swelling, and sometimes redness over the inflamed muscle and tendon structure. Moving it will hurt, and you may be able to feel crepitus as the damaged tendon slides roughly through the irritated tendon sheath. Resting it will feel better.

These symptoms are typical of all kinds of repetitive motion injury. Bikers get it in the knee, hikers in the foot, rowers in the wrists, and writers in the hands. The field treatment is pretty much the same.

Treatment of Tendinitis: You have to break the cycle of injury and inflammation. That is, stop doing what hurts. Easy to say, difficult to do. If possible, splint the limb to minimize the motion of the part that hurts. As pain subsides, remove the splint two or three times a day and do gentle exercises, taking the part through its normal range of motion as pain allows.

Take anti-inflammatory medication like ibuprofen regularly over several days. Apply heat after the initial inflammation has settled down. Use warm soaks four times a day for fifteen minutes at a time. This is good to do just before range of motion exercises.

And . . . how do these fine suggestions help you on day five of a ten-day river trip? Unfortunately, the cause, problem, and symptoms remain the same. You will have to address the treatment differently in order to keep moving.

Change the way you perform the repetitive motion. This will put the stress on different muscle/tendon groups. For example, using a short loop of webbing as a handle on a kayak paddle can allow you to pull with your wrist held vertically instead of horizontally. You won't have the control you're used to, but it may keep you moving.

Take the full therapeutic dose of anti-inflammatory medication. For ibuprofen this is 3,200 mg a day. Your stomach may allow a couple of days of this, which may suppress the inflammation enough to prevent complete disability.

Using tape and padding, you can create a soft splint that will help reduce the stress on the irritated structure. Joint taping is a science in itself, and beyond the scope of this book, but worth learning if you are responsible for kayak, canoe, and hiking groups.

Rest frequently. Let pain be your guide. Stop immediately when the pain begins to grow worse. Continue only after it is under control.

▶ Case Study

S: A twenty-three-year-old female instructor glissading a snow field in the Tetons caught her heel in the snow, causing a tumbling fall. She felt a pop and a brief burning pain in her left knee. On attempting to stand, the knee "gave out." She did not hit her head and has no neck pain. She had full memory for the event. She has an allergy to codeine, takes ibuprofen for headaches, has never injured the knee before, and has no significant past medical history. Her last meal was twenty minutes ago. The glissade was at the end of a ten-day backcountry trip, with only a half mile to go.

O: The instructor was found sitting upright in stable position with the left knee flexed. She was fully alert, warm, and reasonably dry. She had no neck tenderness. The left knee was tender but not swollen, deformed, or discolored. She was able to flex and extend the knee fully with little discomfort. Distal CSM was intact. There was no other obvious injury. Vital signs at 1320 were normal.

A: Unstable injury left knee

A': Distal ischemia due to swelling

P: The knee was splinted with a snowshoe, and an improvised litter was fashioned from ensolite pads and nylon webbing. Despite her embarrassment, the woman was carried the last half mile to the road. Distal CSM was monitored by asking her if she could feel and wiggle her toes inside her boots.

Discussion: Although the temptation to limp the last half mile was very strong, the patient agreed to the appropriate treatment. This injury fit the criteria for unstable injury because of the history of a "pop" during injury and the instability experienced afterward. This story is typical of a ligament rupture.

▶ Case Study

S: A seventeen-year-old girl caught her right index finger between loose rocks during a descent of a scree slope 15 miles from the trailhead. She was able to dislodge herself but complained of immediate pain. Shortly afterward, she became dizzy and nauseous. The group leader climbed back up to examine the girl. Witnesses told him that she did not fall and was not struck by anything. She has no allergies, is not on medication, and has no significant past medical history. She had breakfast one hour ago. She had been walking without difficulty prior to the accident and was well rested and hydrated. The rock was stable but the weather was cool and windy.

O: The patient was found lying against a large rock. She was disoriented, pale, and sweaty. The tip of the right index finger is swollen and very tender with a superficial abrasion of the skin. There was no other injury. Her vital signs at 0930 were BP: unknown, P: 64, R: 24, Skin: pale, cool, moist, T: feels cool, C: V on AVPU with confusion and disorientation, improving.

A: 1. Unstable injury tip of right index finger

    2. Superficial wound

    3. Acute stress reaction

A': 1. Pain and swelling

    2. Infection of abrasion right index finger

P: The finger was immersed in clean, cold water to irrigate the abrasion and relieve pain. She was encouraged to lie in a sleeping bag and calm down. Her vital signs rechecked at 1000 were normal. The finger was splinted by taping it to the third finger with a gauze pad and antibiotic ointment between the fingers.

The girl was instructed to keep the finger elevated as much as possible and use cool soaks for swelling and pain relief during rest stops. The wound was to be irrigated and the dressing changed daily. She was cautioned about the signs and symptoms of infection and instructed to check circulation and sensation at the fingertip frequently. She would be referred to medical care, if necessary, when the group reached the road in three days.

Discussion: Although this patient was displaying very frightening signs and symptoms immediately after the injury, there was no mechanism to explain it except ASR. The changes in mental status rapidly resolved with rest, reassurance, and pain relief, leaving only an unhappy girl with a sore finger. ✚

Musculoskeletal Injury
Wilderness Context

High-Risk Problem:
- Pain out of proportion to the apparent injury
- Critical system injury
- Unstable fracture of pelvis or femur
- Persistent impaired CSM
- Compartment syndrome
- Open fracture
- Joint infection

Chapter 10

Skin and Soft Tissue

In my experience, laceration of the skin was the most common reason that Outward Bound students were evacuated from their solo experience in the Maine islands. The wounds were almost always caused by a slip of the knife blade while rendering some indispensable tool or work of art from a stubborn piece of driftwood. These injuries occur, not for lack of preparation and precaution but rather because the creative spirit seems to get the better of the student's common sense.

To reduce the bloodletting, instructors have used every technique from giving detailed whittling lessons, to "no whittling" policies, to outright banning of knives. But I like the creative spirit and believe the knife to be the most necessary of tools. I tend to favor instruction and precaution and a good talk on wound care.

Students carry into the field with them everything they need to care for minor wounds. This consists of their own two hands, fresh water, soap, and clean gauze dressings. Their primary goal is to assist the body's own defensive and healing mechanisms. Definitive care, such as suturing (stitches), can be performed hours or days later if necessary.

Skin

Epidermis
Dermis

Fat

Fascia

Muscle

STRUCTURE:

- Epidermis/Dermis
- Fat
- Fascia

FUNCTION:

- Thermoregulation
- Sensation
- Fluid retention
- Protection from microbes

PROBLEMS:

- Loss of function due to wounds, burns, or infection

Structure and Function

The skin is the largest of the body's organs. It performs the remarkable function of separating the flora and fauna of the outside environment from the sterile temperature- and chemical-sensitive internal organs. Most of the time it does a pretty good job, considering it's less than a quarter of an inch thick.

The blood vessels in the skin are capable of a dramatic change in volume as they constrict or dilate for thermoregulation or the need to maintain perfusion pressure to the body core. When fully vasodilated, the skin can hold up to 3 liters of blood. When fully vasoconstricted in shell/core effect, the skin may retain as little as 30 milliliters of blood.

Beneath the skin is the soft tissue, consisting of fat, muscle, and connective tissue as well as the small vessels and nerves found in these layers. Problems begin when the protective outer layer of skin is damaged and the soft tissue beneath is exposed. This allows fungi, bacteria, and other creatures to invade unprotected tissue, as well as allowing vital body fluids to escape. Large wounds and burns can cause shock and interfere with the skin's thermoregulatory function.

Wounds

A wound is any injury that disrupts the skin. It can be superficial or deep. All wounds damage blood vessels and cause bleeding. The body can stop this blood loss by automatically constricting blood vessels at the injury site to reduce flow. A clot then begins to form and, if left undisturbed, can bring bleeding to a halt within fifteen minutes.

After the blood loss has been stopped, the slower process of wound repair begins. The initial stages of natural wound cleansing occur over a period of several days. The clot surface dries, forming a natural bandage in the form of a scab. Underlying tissue is further protected by the process of inflammation, which forms a protective barrier below.

Any contamination, such as dirt and bacteria, is moved to the surface as the wound drains. By the third or fourth day, the protective barriers are established and cleansing is well under way. The signs of normal inflammation—redness, warmth, swelling, and pain—begin to subside as the protective barrier continues to grow stronger.

After six to eight days, the wound is very resistant to new outside contamination. As inflammation subsides, wound edges migrate together and form a scar where they meet. Re-injury, or excessive movement or wetting of the wound area, during the early stages can disrupt the barrier effect, allowing infection and delaying healing. This can be a real problem at sea, where staying dry and clean is especially difficult. You must be persistent and creative in protecting a wound in these conditions.

If the protective mechanisms are overwhelmed, invading bacteria can pass through the protective barrier into surrounding tissues. If the body's immune system is unable to control them, bacteria can reproduce rapidly, causing an infection. In an attempt to reestablish the barrier, the body increases local inflammation. Pus develops as the cellular debris and edema fluid accumulates. This combination of processes produces the early signs and symptoms of infection.

If the infection spreads, it will ultimately enter the general circulation and cause a systemic infection, sometimes called blood poisoning. The body responds with systemic inflammation, which produces a generalized redness, fever, and pain. Patients with systemic infection can become very sick. Fortunately, this rarely happens as a complication of skin wounds in healthy people.

Although there are many types of wounds and terms to describe them, we are concerned with the field assessment: simple or high-risk? This is analogous to the stable or unstable assessment of musculoskeletal trauma. Simple wounds offer no risk of life-threatening bleeding and do not represent a significant risk of infection. They can be managed in the field with evacuation to medical care when it is safe to do so.

Simple wounds may involve the skin and subcutaneous fat but do not penetrate into muscle or expose tendons or bone. Simple wounds are clean and free of crushed or dead tissue. A superficial cut from a clean knife is an example.

Some wounds have the potential to cause cosmetic or functional defects as they heal. Examples include wounds of the face, hands, and genitals. You may choose to immediately seek medical care when the risk of evacuation is low because the best cosmetic and functional results will be obtained when wound repair is accomplished within several hours. But this is not worth a high-risk rescue. Acceptable wound repair can be accomplished days later, if necessary.

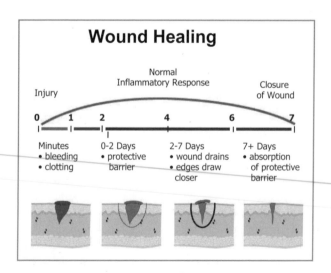

High-risk wounds are those that carry a significant risk of infection or are likely to cause functional problems during early healing. Also labeled as high-risk are wounds associated with life-threatening bleeding or critical system injury. Aggressive field treatment and early evacuation to medical care is ideal.

HIGH-RISK WOUNDS

Grossly Contaminated—Injuries with embedded foreign material, such as gravel, sawdust, or clothing fibers, harbor bacteria that is difficult to dislodge.

Macerated—Wounds in which there is crushed, shredded, or dead tissue that provides growth medium for bacteria.

Deep—Wounds that penetrate the soft tissue to expose joints, tendons, and bones are difficult to clean adequately and are prone to serious infection.

Bites—Mouths harbor a wide variety of virulent bugs. Human bites are among the worst. Cats are pretty bad, too. Any wound exposed to human or animal saliva constitutes a bite wound.

Punctures—A small opening in the skin with a wound track that extends through several layers of tissue deposits bacteria in areas that are unable to drain properly.

Wound assessment is an important skill. Some wounds can appear simple, involving only the skin and fat layers. On closer inspection you may find that deep structures are contaminated. A good field examination may take some time and involve careful probing with an instrument or gloved finger.

Under the skin and fat is a layer of connective tissue called fascia that protects the deep structures underneath. It is easily identified as a tough, dull-white layer of tissue resembling fiberglass. Underlying structures such as tendon, bone, and joint surface appear shiny and white or yellow. Muscle underlying the fascia appears deep red, like a raw steak.

The depth of the wound in millimeters is far less significant than the layers penetrated. An eyelid laceration a few millimeters deep may be high risk while a wound on the buttocks several centimeters deep is considered simple. Puncture wounds often appear very benign on the surface but carry a substantial risk of infection to deep structures. Avulsion flaps should be lifted and inspected for debris and probed for deep structure involvement.

Wounds to the chest or abdomen may enter the organ cavities. There will sometimes be an obvious hollow space, visible or probed. These are very serious and often involve critical system injury. Emergency evacuation to surgical care is lifesaving.

Remember that open wounds also present risk to the examiner. Don't forget to protect your eyes, skin, and mucous membranes from contact with blood and exudates. Wear gloves, eye protection, and keep your mouth shut or wear a mask.

Treatment of Soft Tissue Wounds: Treat the critical body system problems first! Direct pressure stops most bleeding, but to do it effectively you need to see where the blood is coming from. Put on your protective gloves and glasses or goggles and cut away clothes and remove equipment. If pressure is well aimed, most bleeding stops within fifteen minutes as the clotting mechanisms are activated. If bleeding persists, it is usually because the pressure was too light or poorly aimed. Remove the bandage, find the bleeding site, and try again. Once bleeding has stopped, the clot will keep it stopped unless disturbed. Elevation can also help reduce bleeding by reducing the blood pressure in the affected extremity.

A tourniquet can be useful for temporary bleeding control while you are dealing with other critical system problems. It should be applied to the upper arm or thigh using webbing or other wide and soft material. A tourniquet can be left in place for up to an hour with little risk of tissue infarction.

Once bleeding is controlled and your survey for other critical system problems is complete, you are ready to treat a soft tissue wound. There are several steps to follow. These apply to all wounds: big and small, clean and dirty, superficial and deep, and head to toe.

Wound Treatment
WILDERNESS PROTOCOL

Inspect and Clean:

- Clean surrounding skin surface.

- Irrigate with copious amounts of clean water or 1% PI solution.

- Explore wound and remove foreign bodies.

- Cut away dead tissue.

"Proper wound cleaning can take quite a bit of time. Make yourself and your patient comfortable and do a thorough job."

Early wound cleaning will significantly reduce the chance of infection and should be done in the field if evacuation to medical care will take more than two hours. Cleansing a wound usually restarts some bleeding by disturbing the clot. If severe bleeding is a problem, leave the pressure dressing in place until bleeding is definitely stopped. *Do not attempt to clean wounds that are associated with life-threatening bleeding.*

Wash the skin around the wound with soap and water or disinfectant like povidone iodine. Clean a wide area of skin, being careful not to allow soap or disinfectant into the wound itself. Then irrigate the wound with water clean enough to drink. Pour the water directly into the opening and allow it to run out by gravity. The more water, the better. You are flushing out debris and reducing the bacteria count to levels that can be managed by the body's own defenses.

It is unnecessary and harmful to irrigate a wound with full-strength antiseptic preparations like Betadine or peroxide. Antiseptics kill both bacteria and body cells, leaving a partially sterilized wound lined with dead tissue. This can actually *increase* the chances of later infection. If water purification is required, use only a few drops of iodine in a quart of water, as you would to treat it for drinking.

Remove any embedded debris from the wound. Anything that was not flushed out by irrigation should be removed manually. Brush the obvious junk out with a new toothbrush or other clean tool. A pair of tweezers is useful for removing pieces of gravel or clothing that resists gentle persuasion. Cut off any torn pieces of tissue in the wound that are obviously ischemic. These are the pieces of skin and fat that are "hanging by a thread" or have turned blue or black.

Wound Treatment
WILDERNESS PROTOCOL

Remove Impaled Objects Unless:

- Impaled in the globe of the eye
- Removal will cause significant problems:
  - tissue destruction
  - severe bleeding
  - unmanageable pain

An impaled object is best removed by a surgeon in a hospital, but evacuating a patient with an impaled object will often risk more tissue damage than pulling it out. As long as the object remains embedded in the tissue, infection is inevitable. In most cases, impaled objects should be removed in the field and the wounds cleaned like any other. But if it is clear that you are going to do significant damage trying to remove the object, stabilize it in place and evacuate as quickly and carefully as you can. Never remove an impaled object from the globe of the eye. The fluid inside the eye cannot be replaced. Any amount lost will doom the patient's vision.

Properly cleaning a wound can take quite a bit of time, especially if it's very dirty. Go out in the sun or use your head lamp so you can see what you're doing. Make yourself comfortable and take the time to do a good job.

Cover the wound with sterile dressings to prevent contamination. The bandage should not impair circulation or drainage, or prevent wound examination. Meeting these criteria on a wet and dirty expedition can be quite a challenge. Typical first-aid kit adhesive tape and white roller gauze perform poorly in the backcountry or marine environment.

Wound Treatment
WILDERNESS PROTOCOL

<u>High-Risk Wound Care:</u>

- Clean as with any other wound unless there is risk of life-threatening bleeding

- Early evacuation

- Consider antibiotics if authorized

- Contact local health department about rabies risk in mammal bites

"Gentle probing with a sterilized instrument or gloved finger may reveal a previously unnoticed laceration of the fascia exposing muscle or joint space to contamination."

Newer dressings designed for long-term care of open wounds and stasis ulcers offer the medical officer some good options for backcountry use. A sterile, transparent, semipermeable membrane can be left in place for several days. Semipermeable membranes are also combined with colloidal dressings to absorb drainage, keep the wound moist, and prevent external contamination even in very wet and dirty situations. The dressings are expensive but far superior to the standard-issue first-aid supplies.

An inexpensive roller bandage known as "vet wrap," originally developed for veterinary use, can be used for splints or to hold dressings in place far more effectively than tape or elastic wrap. It is water resistant, self-amalgamating, and reusable. Abrasions and shallow wounds in which only the superficial layers of skin are affected can be dressed with antibiotic ointment alone, or with an easily removed sterile dressing. Because the most common anticipated problem with abrasions is infection, frequent cleaning and inspection is a priority. Antibiotic ointment can also be used alone in difficult-to-bandage places such as eyelids and ears.

Leaving the wound open and allowing it to drain is important. Do not pull the wound edges together with tape or try to suture it with your dental floss. Closing a wound in the field is likely to create a nice demonstration of the Obstruction to Infection principle!

Splint the extremity if the wound is over a joint or in another area of skin that is mobile. This will minimize the breakdown of the protective barrier. Unless it restricts travel, it will also make the patient more comfortable.

High-risk wounds should receive early medical attention whenever possible, especially where open fracture is suspected. Infection generally takes a day or two to get going, so your ideal evacuation plan would have your patient out of the woods within forty-eight hours. During your walk out, the wound should receive the same careful attention as any other. This is especially true for the removal of debris and irrigation. If your treatment is particularly effective, infection may never start.

Antibiotics given immediately offer some protection against the development of infection in high-risk wounds. If you are sailing or trekking days from medical care, carrying these drugs is a reasonable precaution. You should obtain a prescription and instructions from a medical practitioner.

Sutures or staples are used mainly to connect deep structures, such as tendons and ligaments, and to close gaping wounds to reduce healing time and minimize scarring. Closing a wound requires training, experience, and a scrupulously clean environment. In the majority of cases, it is not necessary or appropriate as a field treatment. The kind of simple wound that might be successfully sutured by an inexperienced person doesn't need it anyway. Deep or complicated wounds need professional attention and should not be repaired by amateurs. Unless you really know what you are doing, leave the suture kit at home. Wound repair or scar revision can be safely delayed for days or weeks if necessary.

Tetanus prophylaxis is an injectable vaccine given to anyone with an open wound who has not had a vaccination within ten years, or five years with particularly dirty wounds. This is best done within twenty-four hours of injury. You can keep this from becoming a problem by keeping your routine tetanus vaccinations up to date.

Monitor the wound and your patient for signs of infection whether or not you choose to evacuate. You should also monitor distal CSM as you would with a musculoskeletal problem. Bandages, splints, and swelling can create the same ischemia here as well.

Wound Infection

Infection is a possibility in any wound at any time during the healing process, but it is most likely to appear within two to four days after injury. It takes about that long for the typical skin surface bacteria that has invaded the deeper layers to multiply and do enough damage to produce inflammation. But this time frame can vary widely depending on the health of the individual, virulence of the bacteria, and quality of wound care.

In normal wound healing, pain, swelling, redness, and inflammation decrease quickly within the first two or three days. If the wound becomes infected, these signs and symptoms will begin to increase instead. Pus may be seen in the wound and be accompanied by a foul odor.

If the symptoms affect only the immediate area of the wound, the infection is considered local. When bacteria begin to spread beyond the wound into the rest of the body, it is considered systemic. The signs and symptoms of systemic infection include fever, nausea, generalized swelling of a larger area around the wound, and red streaks running toward the heart from the site of infection.

Wound Infection

Local Infection:

- Increasing redness, pain, warmth, swelling
- Most likely to develop days 2 - 4
- Drainage or accumulation of pus (abscess)

Systemic Infection:

- Fever, malaise, regional swelling
- Lymphangitis (red streaks)
- Vascular and volume shock

Treatment of Wound Infection: Almost any wound that is becoming infected earns the status of "high risk" and should receive medical care. En route, you should continue regular cleaning and dressing changes. If the infected wound has been closed with tape or sutures, it should be opened and allowed to drain. Irrigate with water to remove pus. Do not squeeze an infected wound or you will just drive bacteria through the protective barrier into healthy tissues.

If an abscess has formed close to the skin surface, it can be safely opened with a sharp knife, irrigated, and allowed to drain. Clean the skin surface with antiseptic or soap and nick the pus pocket with a sterile blade. This procedure is reserved for those cases where the pus pocket is obvious and superficial. Don't attempt to incise anything in the deeper layers of soft tissue.

Heat applications will increase circulation to the area to help the body fight the infection locally. Use only as much heat as you can comfortably stand against normal skin. Apply for thirty minutes at a time as often as five to six times a day.

Systemic infection is a medical emergency. Antibiotics should be started immediately, preferably by injection. Urgent evacuation is required. Septic shock, which is a form of vascular shock, is an anticipated problem.

Burns

All burns are caused by heat transmitted from hot gases or objects, or produced by a chemical reaction between the skin and a caustic substance. Burns can involve internal structures, such as the respiratory system, as well as the outside skin.

For field management, we need to know the depth and extent of burns as well as location. The extent is described in terms of body surface area (BSA), and critical locations include hands, feet, genitalia, and the respiratory system.

Estimates of irregular burns can be made using the size of one surface of the patient's hand, which is about 1 percent of the body surface area. The depth of burn refers to how deep the damage goes. This can be difficult to estimate, particularly where different areas are burned to various degrees.

PARTIAL-THICKNESS BURNS

First Degree: The skin integrity is not disrupted. Capillaries and nerves are intact. Inflammation occurs normally with redness, pain, and warmth. This is the typical sunburn.

Second Degree: The skin surface is damaged, but the injury is limited to outer layers. Capillaries are damaged, but deeper skin blood vessels and nerves are intact, allowing inflammation to produce blisters. There is fluid loss, redness, warmth, and pain.

FULL-THICKNESS BURNS

Third Degree: The full thickness of skin is damaged. Capillaries, blood vessels, and nerves are destroyed. Normal inflammation cannot occur, and as a result, blisters do not develop. The burned area may appear charred black or gray. The area may not be painful due to loss of nerves. Small third-degree burns may appear to be less serious because of this.

As with other injury, look first for potentially life-threatening problems. These will usually come in the form of volume shock and/or respiratory distress. High-risk burns are those that are likely to involve significant anticipated problems due to the potential for critical body system involvement, pain, infection, or scar formation.

HIGH-RISK BURNS

Any respiratory system involvement: Burned respiratory passages will develop the same inflammation, blisters, and fluid loss that are seen on the skin. Signs and symptoms include singed facial hair, burned lips, sooty sputum, and persistent cough.

Respiratory distress may develop from pulmonary edema or from swelling and obstruction in the airways. As with any other swelling, it can develop quickly or slowly over a period of hours. Respiratory burns carry a mortality rate of about 20 percent.

Partial-thickness burns of the face, genitalia, and hands: Any significant burns in these areas can cause problems with swelling and ischemia in the short term, and mobility and scarring in the long term.

Burns of any degree greater than 10 percent BSA: Large burns carry the anticipated problem of volume shock and hypothermia.

Any full-thickness burn: Any full-thickness burn is at high risk for infection.

Chemical burns: It can be difficult to fully arrest the burning process as some chemicals react with the skin. Damage can continue for hours afterward.

Electrical burns: Skin damage may be minor, but AC electrical current can cause extensive injury to internal organs and tissues. Lightning tends to cause only superficial burns and little internal electrical injury.

Burns of very young or very old patients

Burns

Treatment:

- Immediate cooling.
- Continue cooling for several minutes.
- Irrigate with water or 1% PI solution.
- Remove dead skin.
- Decompress blisters only if necessary.
- Dress to prevent contamination.
- Monitor for infection.

Treatment of Burns: Stop the burning process. The first step in the management of burns is to immediately remove the heat. The fastest way to do this is to immerse the patient or injured part in water. Fortunately, this is almost instinctive, as it serves to relieve pain as well. Be careful, as it is possible with larger burns to make your patient hypothermic as a side effect of your good intentions. If the burn is greater than about 10 percent body surface area, limit your cooling to only a few minutes. In chemical burns continued irrigation with water will not only cool the area but also help remove the chemical itself. Irrigation should continue for at least thirty minutes.

Dressing a large surface area burn can be difficult. The goal is to minimize contamination and reduce evaporative cooling. An improvised dressing can consist of a clean cotton T-shirt covered with a waterproof clothing layer. Plastic kitchen wrap will also work. Immediate attention should be given to maintaining hydration and body core temperature. The patient will need food, fluids, and protection during evacuation. Prophylactic antibiotics may be indicated for large or contaminated burns. There is some evidence that ibuprofen can reduce the inflammation and long-term damage from sunburn. Aloe vera gel is useful to relieve pain and provide some topical antibiotic and anti-inflammatory effect.

If burns have the potential to cause life-threatening critical body system problems, use basic life support techniques and plan an emergency evacuation. With large burns, respiratory distress and shock are common. Any respiratory burn should be carefully monitored and evacuated without waiting for the development of severe symptoms.

Even a sunburn can be a significant problem in the wilderness setting if it occupies a large area of skin surface. Ultraviolet radiation causes inflammation of the dermis and epidermis, inhibiting skin function and causing pain and redness.

You should anticipate all of the same problems inherent in any large surface area burn: volume shock, thermoregulatory problems, pain, and infection.

If the burn is not a life-threatening emergency, clean and dress it with antibiotic dressings like minor abrasion. This can be done along with the application of cool soaks for pain relief. Continue to treat as any open wound. If the burn falls under the category of "high risk," plan to have the patient to medical care within about forty-eight hours if possible.

Burn Treatment

Non-stick dressings:

- Xeroform or petroleum gauze
- Plastic wrap
- Gel dressings

Anticipate:

- Hypothermia in large burns
- Volume shock in large burns
- Infection in partial or full thickness burns

Wounds and Burns
Wilderness Context

High Risk Problem:

- Large surface area burns
- Systemic infection (lymphangitis, fever)
- Pain out of proportion to apparent injury
- Uncontrolled bleeding or fluid loss
- Respiratory involvement in burn
- Rapidly progressing local infection.
- Distal ischemia.

Blisters

Blisters, like the kind you get on your feet while hiking, are really burns caused by the heat generated by friction. Your boots and socks rub against your skin and the damage results in leaky capillaries and swelling, and there you are. You not only have a skin injury to treat but a transportation problem as well. Keep walking on it and you will need a ride out of the woods just as surely as if you'd broken your leg.

Blisters progress through three stages. They begin with "hot spots," progress to blisters filled with sterile fluid, and then break to become contaminated superficial wounds. The stage at which you confront them, and your logistical situation, will determine your treatment. Generally, they act just like other "shallow wounds."

Treatment of Blisters: Hot spots are when you begin to feel discomfort. You know something is wrong in your left boot, but you're only ten minutes into the hike and you don't want to stop yet. I don't blame you, especially if the black flies are bad. But stop you must. Outward Bound instructors routinely stop their group early in their first hike to do a foot check and a talk on blister prevention.

Stop the friction now, and you can prevent a blister from forming. Change your socks, fiddle with your laces, or cover the sore area with smooth surface tape, gel dressings, or mole skin. You can also apply antibiotic ointment to lubricate the area and reduce friction. Whatever time it takes to cool the hot spot will be well worth it in the long run, and save you from . . .

Blisters that you can't always avoid. The important fact to remember early on is that a blister is a sterile wound until it breaks. Whenever we can, we like to keep it that way. Like an abrasion, the lower layers of the skin are still intact, so the wound will heal quickly from below. Small blisters can be covered with gel dressing. Larger ones will usually cause some degree of disability unless you can take the pressure off.

Blisters

Prevent Friction and Heat:

- Moleskin, donut dressing

- Smooth tape

- Gel dressings

Treatment:

- Unroof blister if it appears infected.

- Drain blister if it prevents travel.

- Dress as partial thickness burn.

If the blister has formed in a bad spot, like the back of your heel, you may have to drain it in order to be able to walk. You will be converting a closed and sterile wound into an open one. We can minimize the risk of infection by treating the wound before it happens.

As with other wounds, clean the skin around and over the blister with soap and water. Sterilize a needle or sharp knife blade by flame or alcohol. Make a tiny hole in the blister at the lower margin and allow the fluid to drain out. Leave the skin over the blister intact to act as its own sterile dressing. Cover the area with antibiotic ointment and dress it as you might a "hot spot." Like any open wound, it must be cleaned and dressed daily and monitored for signs of infection.

Open blisters occur when a blister has broken into a non-sterile environment. It should be treated like an abrasion. Cut away the dead skin and irrigate to remove debris, then cover the wound with antibiotic ointment and sterile dressings. Clean daily and monitor for infection. Fix the source of friction with padding or tape.

▶ Case Study

S: A twenty-three-year-old student on a research vessel was struck on the head by a swinging davit when a winch cable snapped. He was found sitting on deck with a large and freely bleeding laceration across the top of his head.

He remembered everything about the event. He denied neck pain and has no other complaints. He denied allergies, was taking no medications, was well fed and warm, had no significant medical history, and was up to date on his tetanus vaccination.

The vessel was in the Gulf Stream approximately 300 miles southeast of Cape Cod. The weather was mild but expected to deteriorate over the next twenty-four hours.

O: Awake and oriented, cooperative, holding a blood-soaked kerchief on his head. Blood covered his left shoulder and chest, and there was a large pool on the deck. He has no neck deformity or tenderness, has full range of motion and normal sensation of the extremities with no numbness or tingling. The scalp had a 4 cm laceration, clean and straight, through the skin and subcutaneous tissue to the skull. No depression or bone fragments can be seen or felt. Vital signs at 1805 were BP: 112/78, P: 88, R: 16, C: Awake and oriented, T: normal, Skin: normal color and temperature.

A: 1. Scalp wound

A': Wound infection (unlikely)

P: 1. Direct pressure to stop bleeding. Clean surrounding scalp and hair with soap and water. Irrigate wound with water. Dress with sterile dressings and a hat to hold them in place. Monitor and redress twice a day. Follow up with physician in Bermuda during planned port call in three days.

Discussion: The scalp did just what it was designed to do. By slipping and tearing, it absorbed enough of the force of the impact to protect the skull and brain. There was no brain injury, just a scalp wound. As is common to the scalp, bleeding was profuse but easily controlled with direct pressure. Although it looked like a lot of blood, vital signs show that not enough was lost to produce shock. Because of the rich blood supply, even deep scalp wounds usually heal well with a very low incidence of infection. There was no emergency here.

Unfortunately, bloody scalp wounds generate a lot of unnecessary anxiety and precipitate a lot of dangerous evacuations. Coast Guard and Navy records are full of long flights in bad weather to rescue patients just like this one. Whatever benefit this might have must be weighed against sometimes substantial risks. If you think that *your* life is exciting, talk to a helicopter pilot about in-flight refueling at night. ✚

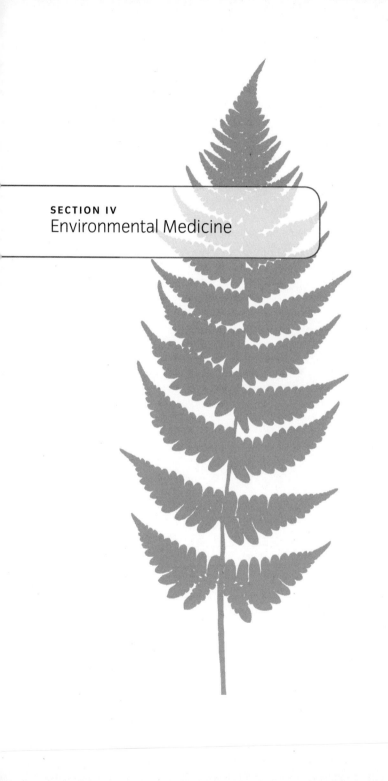

SECTION IV
Environmental Medicine

Toxic substances can produce systemic effects, local effects, or both. Toxins, like trauma, can cause simultaneous involvement of more than one body system. The cause-and-effect relationship may be fairly obvious or quite confusing.

A toxin can also cause an allergic reaction, further complicating the picture. A hornet sting is an example of a substance that can do both. Fortunately, a toxic reaction is not often mixed with allergy even though the type of exposure and symptoms may be similar.

Systemic toxins are those that affect the body as a whole. They may be ingested, injected, inhaled, or absorbed through the skin. Some common examples include mushrooms, cobra venom, and carbon monoxide. These can be immediately life-threatening, or the onset of symptoms can be delayed by many hours.

Local toxins affect only the immediate area of body contact. The toxin in a tarantula bite does not significantly affect critical body systems but may cause localized tissue swelling and pain. Some toxins have both systemic and local effects. An example would be an inhaled gas that irritates the respiratory system while being absorbed through the lungs into the general circulation.

When you are not sure exactly what you're dealing with, base your emergency treatment on what you see and environmental conditions around you. Don't worry so much about identifying the toxin that you forget to treat the patient. Support critical body systems and treat anaphylaxis if you see it. Maintain body core temperature and hydration, and provide pain relief.

Any toxin causing respiratory distress, shock, altered mental status, or severe pain represents an emergency. Begin planning an immediate evacuation. You still may not know exactly what the toxin is, but you will be supporting life functions and moving in the right direction.

Treatment of Ingested Toxins

A brief review of anatomy reminds us that an ingested substance does not actually enter the body until it is absorbed by the lining of the digestive system. A glass marble swallowed by a child will not be absorbed and will pass harmlessly through the gut. This is the goal for treatment of an ingested toxin, too.

When one of your young and adventurous clients decides to sample the local mushrooms, try to dilute the toxin and reduce its absorption using lots of water and activated charcoal. At a dose of 25 to 50 grams orally, activated charcoal may bind some of the substances in the gut, helping to prevent absorption through the mucus membranes in the intestine. Even if it does not help with a specific toxin, it will cause no harm. Water will move the substance through the gut more quickly on its way to excretion.

Effective antidotes to toxins are not always available. Certainly their use is limited to cases where the toxin is known, such as certain drugs and plants. If possible, contact a poison control center or local medical facility for specific treatments. The availability of an antidote in one place or another may influence your evacuation decisions. In any case most toxins are excreted or metabolized by the body over hours or days.

Drug overdose is another common source of ingested toxin. You should know the risks associated with overdose of any drug that you carry in quantity. The likely source of a problem will be overuse of pain medication like acetaminophen, ibuprofen, or narcotics like hydrocodone. This can happen when patients are confused about generic and trade names used for drugs. For example, a patient may take full doses of two different brands of pain reliever, hoping for a better result, not realizing that both are trade names for the same acetaminophen. The effects of a mild unintentional overdose are usually limited to accentuated side effects like stomach upset or drowsiness. Discontinuing the medication usually solves the problem.

Intentional overdose is another matter. Even common over-the-counter medications such as acetaminophen or iron tablets can be toxic in high doses. Immediate generic treatment followed by emergency evacuation is indicated. In narcotic or antihistamine overdose, the immediate threat to life will be respiratory failure due to loss of respiratory drive. Oxygen and positive pressure ventilation can be lifesaving.

Food poisoning is another form of accidental toxic ingestion. The toxin is produced by bacteria such as staphylococci growing in or on poorly refrigerated food. The bacteria are usually destroyed by stomach acid or cooking, but the toxin survives to be absorbed by the gut. Symptoms are usually limited to gastrointestinal upset including cramps, diarrhea, and vomiting. The disease is self-limiting, and the primary anticipated problem is shock from dehydration. Hydration is the primary treatment.

Food poisoning is differentiated from bacterial infection of the gut by the absence of fever or blood and pus in diarrhea, and usually resolves within twenty-four hours. You should suspect infection in any gastrointestinal illness that lasts longer than that. A bacterial infection of the gut should be considered serious and aggressively treated with antibiotics and evacuation.

It may be impossible to distinguish between a mild gastroenteritis caused by a viral infection and food poisoning because the signs and symptoms are often the same. Your primary clue will be the mechanism of injury. You should suspect food poisoning when a number of people who ate the same meal develop the same symptoms.

Ciguterra and scombroid, toxins ingested with food, are worthy of special mention for the marine environment. Cigutoxin is produced by a reef-dwelling dynoflagellate that is consumed by coral and other reef animals. It is concentrated up the food chain, reaching dangerous levels in larger predatory fish. It produces gastrointestinal symptoms as well as neurologic symptoms such as numbness, tingling, cramping, and reversal of hot and cold sensation that may persist for months. Ciguterra toxin can be avoided by restricting your hunting to fish smaller than a kilogram or so.

Scombroid toxin is a histamine-like substance produced by bacteria growing on the surface of dead fish in storage. Scombroid produces a histamine-like response, including hives, itching, and flushed skin. It can be difficult to distinguish from an allergic reaction. Fortunately, the treatment is the same.

Symptoms developing after consumption of fish and shellfish should be treated like any other ingested toxin. Water and activated charcoal will help dilute and remove the toxin, minimizing absorption by the gut. Hives and itching can be effectively treated with an antihistamine like diphenhydramine. Persistent or severe neurological symptoms should be evacuated to medical care.

Treatment of Absorbed Toxins

Clean the exposed area as you would for any skin wound. Start by irrigating with lots of water. Removal of some substances may require a different solvent capable of cutting waxy or oily compounds. Alcohol, vinegar, and even WD-40 have found a place in initial treatment. Check with local medical facilities for recommendation on treating exposure to poisonous plants, preferably before the exposure occurs. The sap of the manchineel tree found throughout the tropics is a good example. Blisters should be left intact. Topical steroid creams may be helpful for superficial inflammation. Antibiotic ointment may help prevent infection.

Remember that the toxin may still be present on clothing and equipment that could come into contact with the patient or other members of the group. Some toxins like manchineel sap (*Hippomane mancinella*) will continue to spread on clothing and skin until completely removed. Clean your gear thoroughly to avoid perpetuating the problem.

As with large burns or abrasions, the surface area involved can lead to serious problems with even superficial injury. Large surface area inflammation can lead to dehydration, infection, and hypothermia. Any serious involvement of more than about 10 percent of body surface area should be considered high risk. Be alert to respiratory involvement that carries the anticipated problem of respiratory distress and failure.

Surface Absorbed

Treatment:

- BLS, PROP
- Remove and dilute: brush off or irrigate with water
- Dress open wounds, burns, and blisters. BSA >10% is high risk
- Evacuate with ALS assistance as needed.
- Contact poison control

Eg: Manchineeal sap, insect repellants, organophosphate fertilizers.

Treatment of Inhaled Toxins

Toxic inhalation can cause problems through two distinct mechanisms. Inhaled substances can be absorbed through the lungs into the body or cause direct respiratory system injury. Carbon monoxide poisoning from using a heater or stove inside a poorly vented snow cave is an example of the former, and chlorine gas is an example of the latter.

Carbon monoxide gas causes no direct respiratory system injury but prevents oxygen from being absorbed into the blood. The patient quietly asphyxiates and the problem may go unnoticed until it is too late. Like most inhaled toxins, the treatment is ventilation and fresh air. If instituted soon enough, there should be no lasting damage to critical body systems, including the respiratory system.

Direct injury can be caused by the inhalation of caustic substances. Chlorine gas directly damages the respiratory system. Symptoms include inflammation around the nose and mouth, coughing, wheezing, burning chest pain, and respiratory distress. Early recognition and treatment of respiratory distress is the key to survival. Identifying the specific toxin in these cases is not as important as emergency field treatment and evacuation.

Inhaled Toxins

Treatment:

- BLS, PROP
- Remove and dilute: PPV, fresh air and oxygen
- Respiratory system injury is high risk
- Evacuate with ALS assistance as needed
- Contact poison control

Eg: Carbon monoxide, cooking and heating gas, volcanic gases.

Treatment of Injected Toxins: Bites and Stings

Toxins used by animals while hunting or defending themselves come in two basic types: neurotoxins and tissue toxins. Neurotoxins interfere with the function of the nervous system, causing muscle spasm, paralysis, and altered sensation. In rare fatal cases the cause of death is usually respiratory failure due to paralysis of the breathing muscles.

Tissue toxins destroy body cells, causing inflammation, pain, and swelling. Damage is usually localized with distal ischemia and infection as anticipated problems. Severe envenomations can also produce systemic effects and multiorgan failure and volume shock. Fortunately, this is rare.

Many animals use a combination of tissue toxin and neurotoxin to subdue their prey. Antidotes are available to the toxins of some specific organisms, and to some groups of similar species. If you are traveling off the beaten path, it is well worth research into toxic species and the availability and location of antivenin.

The vast majority of stings and bites are no more significant than the minimal discomfort that they cause. The few that are significant are easily identified by severe pain, swelling, or the progression of neurological symptoms. The important principle of field treatment for significant envenomations is to provide good basic life support while moving toward the appropriate definitive medical care. The identification of the specific species encountered can be valuable in planning treatment if medical facilities are accessible, but it should not delay evacuation.

Marine Bites and Stings: In the marine environment, toxin is most commonly infiltrated by spines or injected by nematocysts. They range in potency from the merely annoying to the rapidly fatal. Again, the recognition of species is not as important as the recognition and treatment of a critical system problem.

Spines are used for defense, and some of these are coated with toxins. Examples include stingrays, scorpion fish, catfish, and some sea urchins. The species found in waters around North America generally produce only the localized pain and swelling of tissue toxins. In Indo-Pacific waters the organisms can be more dangerous, carrying significant neurotoxic effects as well. The cone shell and box jelly are two notable examples.

The sting of a poisonous ray, urchin, or fish is easy to distinguish from a non-toxic puncture. The pain caused by the wound itself is minimal compared to the quickly increasing discomfort caused by the toxin, which may possess both tissue toxic and neurotoxic characteristics. The barbed stinger or spine will often remain in the wound. Because the spine may be coated with a sheath of tissue that contaminates the wound, infection is likely.

Treatment of Spiny Envenomation: Treatment includes removal of the spine or stinger and aggressive wound debridement. Because many types of spiny toxins are inactivated by heat, immerse the affected part in water as hot as the patient can tolerate until pain is relieved. Often this will be within a few minutes.

Spiny Injury

Treatment:

- Immerse extremity in hot water up to 90 minutes

- High-risk wound care, anticipate infection

- BLS/ALS and immediate evacuation for progressive neurologic symptoms (lionfish, stonefish, cone shell)

- Pain control

Typically tissue toxin, sometimes combined with neurotoxin

The other major hunting tools used by marine organisms are nematocysts. These are the tiny structures in the stinging parts of jellyfish, corals, and anemones that fire something resembling a microscopic harpoon when touched. These harpoons then inject a potent neurotoxin into the skin of the prey. Individually the amount of toxin is miniscule, but the toxin load can be considerable when thousands of nematocysts fire at once. The unlucky fish or other creature, now paralyzed, floats into the digestive organ of the hunter to become its next meal.

Fortunately for us we are not going to become a meal for a jellyfish or anemone. We're too big and we probably taste bad. While the toxin load can paralyze a small fish, it is usually just annoying and painful to something the size of a human. Notable exceptions include stings from the Indo-Pacific box jellyfish (the most dangerous is Chironex fleckeri), due to the high potency of the venom, and the Portuguese man-of-war, due to the potential for large surface area exposure.

Nematocyst Injury

Treatment:

- Rinse with salt water, remove tentacles
- Vinegar soaks (most species)
- General wound care, topical corticosteroids
- BLS/ALS and immediate evacuation for progressive neurologic symptoms (box jelly, man-of-war)
- Pain control

Typically neurotoxic effects with skin inflammation

Treatment of Nematocyst Stings: The general field treatment for stinging jellyfish includes removing tentacles by flushing with seawater and picking off any remaining tentacles with forceps or gloved fingers. Seawater is thought to be preferable to fresh water because the osmotic difference of fresh water may stimulate more nematocysts to fire. Flushing and soaking the skin with vinegar will inactivate the nematocysts of some species and is specifically recommended for box jellyfish, fireworm, and sponge stings. Ice applications may help relieve the pain. The use of alcohol, meat tenderizer, urine, or other chemicals to flush the skin is not helpful and possibly harmful.

Persistent skin inflammation can be treated for several days with twice-daily applications of a steroid cream or ointment like those containing hydrocortisone. Antihistamines may also help because allergic reaction may be a component of the patient's discomfort. As with any open wound, infection is an anticipated problem, and good wound care is important.

Systemic effects from large or potent exposure to nematocyst-borne neurotoxins include pain, spasm, and cramping. Medical follow-up is recommended for any exposure that produces significant systemic symptoms. An exposure occupying more than 50 percent of a limb should also be considered potentially serious.

Truly life-threatening symptoms are very rare and generally limited to patients exposed to the Portugese man-of-war and the Indo-Pacific box jellyfish. Box jellyfish venom can produce cardiac arrhythmia, respiratory paralysis, and a dangerous elevation of blood pressure. For this reason, antivenin to this toxin is carried and administered in the field by rescue personnel in high-incidence areas of Australia and Southeast Asia. Basic life support and immediate evacuation are indicated. Consult local authorities about the area you plan to operate in.

There is no antivenin for the Portuguese man-of-war. Fortunately, fatalities from exposure are very rare. Symptoms include severe burning sensations and skin erythema, which tends to disappear within an hour. Initial treatment includes only flushing with water and removal of tentacles, and treatment for pain. Vinegar is not recommended for this exposure.

More significant exposure to the Portuguese man-of-war can cause muscle cramping, temporary numbness and weakness in the area of exposure, and lymph node swelling. Allergic reactions are uncommon, but you should be alert to the signs and symptoms of anaphylaxis mixed with the toxic effects. Any persistent or severe symptoms require follow-up medical care.

Poisonous Snakes

In North America there are two types of poisonous snakes, pit vipers and coral snakes. The pit vipers include rattlesnakes, copperheads, and cottonmouths. Pit viper venom is primarily a tissue toxin that causes local swelling and tissue damage. Systemic effects include problems with blood coagulation and shock caused by leakage of fluid from the circulatory system into the interstitial space (between the cells in body tissues). Some pit viper venom, notably the Mojave rattlesnake, also contains a systemic neurotoxin. The degree of systemic effect depends on the dose injected and the size and general health of the patient. Fatalities in North America are extremely rare.

While pit viper venom is mostly tissue toxic, coral snake venom is neurotoxic. The fangs of the coral snake are quite small so the snake will have to chew its way into your skin to successfully inject venom. It requires handling of the snake to be bitten. The victims are usually children or intoxicated teenage males. The venom's effects may be delayed for several hours.

Symptoms of coral snake bite include tingling of the extremity, possibly progressing to the whole body. Fatalities due to respiratory failure are also extremely rare.

Treatment of Poisonous Snakebite: The specific and ideal treatment for poisonous snakebite is antivenin. Because pit viper antivenin is the same for all of the members of that family of snakes, it is not necessary to know the difference between a rattlesnake, copperhead, or cottonmouth. The presence of fang marks is enough. Coral snake antivenin is distinct. Fortunately, a coral snake is easily distinguished from a pit viper.

Evacuation to medical care should be started without delay by the fastest means available. Walking your patient out to the trailhead to meet the ambulance may be the quickest way to go, and this is fine unless severe symptoms prevent it. If possible, alert the hospital to expect your patient so that antivenin can be acquired and prepared. The use of antivenin is restricted to the hospital because it can cause life-threatening allergic reactions in rare cases.

Splinting the bitten extremity may help reduce pain and tissue damage but is an unproven treatment and should not delay evacuation. Do not apply ice or arterial or venous tourniquets or use electric shock devices. Do not apply suction devices or cut into the wound. None of these treatments have been shown to be particularly effective and may be harmful if improperly applied.

In anticipation of swelling, remove constricting items such as rings, bracelets, and tight clothing to prevent ischemia. Closely monitor any splint for the same reason. If you can, mark the progression of swelling up the extremity. Make a line and write the time on the skin with a pen. This information will be helpful to the hospital personnel in the use of antivenin.

In parts of the world outside of North America, fang-bearing snakes possess more destructive forms of venom. The use of lymphatic compression bandages is sometimes employed with snakebites that contain more potent neurotoxins. It is worth research into the types of snakes, recommended treatments and location of antivenin for the region in which you will be traveling. You may find, for example, that the nearest antivenin for the poisonous Fer de Lance in Trinidad is actually in Miami. Check before you need it.

Pit Viper Envenomation

Treatment:

- Evacuate to antivenom!
- Anticipate swelling
- Splint extremity if it will not delay evacuation
- NO tourniquets, ice, suction devices!
- IV hydration if available
- BLS

Insects and Arachnids

Insect and arachnid venom is injected by a stinger or specialized mouthparts as the animal attempts to defend itself or warn you away from a nest. It is meant to hurt, and it usually does. This is typical of wasps, fire ants, spiders, and scorpions.

More commonly, your skin reacts to the irritation of substances used by a feeding insect to prevent clotting of your blood. Many of them also inject a local anesthetic to reduce the pain caused by the bite, at least for as long as they're feeding. Examples of these insects include blackflies, moose flies, mosquitoes, no-see-ums, and most of the fauna of North America.

Local reaction to toxins can be severe but involve only the extremity or immediate area of the bite or sting. There may be some degree of acute stress reaction that must be distinguished from systemic effects. Local reactions are treated for comfort. Use cool soaks, elevation, and rest. Aspirin, ibuprofen, or other anti-inflammatory pain medications will help, as will diphenhydramine or other antihistamines.

Toxin load is the term applied to the cumulative effects of multiple stings or bites. The effects can be immediate, as with a large number of bee stings, or delayed up to twenty-four hours. Delayed reactions are common in blackfly country in the spring and early summer. Symptoms include fever, fatigue, headache, and nausea. This is not an allergic reaction if the generalized swelling, respiratory distress, and other signs of anaphylaxis are absent.

This is usually not a major critical system problem. Observe for twenty-four hours. Give aspirin, ibuprofen, or other anti-inflammatory pain reliever for comfort. Watch for signs of infection at the site of insect bites. Keep the patient well hydrated and protected from excessive cooling or heating. They will not be happy, but they will get better.

BLACK WIDOW

The black widow (*Latrodectus mactans*), found in the warmer parts of the United States and farther south, uses a potent neurotoxin to immobilize insect prey. Biting a human is purely defensive; they are not feeding on you. The spider prefers dark and quiet places, so people are bitten most often when reaching into dark and quiet spaces or sitting on an outhouse seat. The bite itself is only mildly uncomfortable.

The symptoms of black widow envenomation develop later and include muscle cramping (especially in the abdomen), pain, and numbness and muscle weakness. The development of these symptoms shortly after crawling around likely habitat should raise the suspicion of a black widow bite. Treatment includes evacuation to medical care because your patient may require critical system support and medication to reduce muscle spasm. Antivenin is available but may carry more risk than the venom itself. Symptoms usually resolve over several days. In spite of its ominous name, death from the bite of a black widow is very rare.

BROWN RECLUSE

The brown recluse is a large spider found in the southeast United States that injects a long-acting tissue toxin causing localized tissue inflammation and necrosis. The initial bite may go unnoticed, with a pustule developing several days later. This is often mistaken for an infection caused by a splinter or other foreign body. It does not respond to incision and drainage or antibiotics. The lesion can continue to progress over days and weeks to involve a large area of tissue destruction, which may become secondarily infected. A suspected brown recluse bite should be referred to a surgeon.

SCORPIONS

Most scorpion stings are described as similar to or a bit worse than your average wasp. Most annoying in North America is the *Centroidies excilicauda,* which employs a potent neurotoxin. Pain may last for hours to days. There is no specific field treatment beyond pain medication. Ice is not indicated. Significant systemic symptoms are rare and include agitation and respiratory paralysis, and should prompt an evacuation to medical care. An antivenin is available but is a high-risk treatment due to the incidence of serum sickness and anaphylaxis. No fatalities from *Centroidies* stings have been reported in the United States, but the animal's venom is more potent in Central and South America.

TICKS

The saliva of some species of ticks contains a neurotoxin capable of causing symptoms in humans, most commonly in children. Tick paralysis can develop after four or more days of attachment and is characterized by numbness and paralysis progressing up the legs and arms. The patient may exhibit a stumbling gait, restlessness, or irritability. The diagnosis is suspected by finding an engorged tick and confirmed by rapid improvement following removal of the tick.

Tick paralysis is rare. Ticks are more commonly implicated as vectors of disease. Prevention of tick paralysis and tick-borne disease depends on avoiding bites and early removal of attached ticks.

▶ **Case Study: Toxins**

S: An eighteen-year-old male on a spring break canoe trip on Lake Powell was bitten on the left forearm by a 4-foot snake that he was attempting to capture and bring back to camp. In the ensuing confusion, the snake escaped. The man was unable to describe it other than being dark in color and very fast. He complained of pain in the mid left forearm and of feeling very faint.

It was early evening, the sky was clear, and the temperature was about 70 degrees. The camp was located approximately 7 miles from the marina at Bullfrog. In spite of a stiff headwind on the lake, the patient was carried to a canoe for evacuation to the marina. Unfortunately, the paddlers were also intoxicated and became lost in the darkness. They returned to camp two hours later, unsure of where they had been.

The patient was reevaluated by a wilderness first responder who had not been drinking. The patient, now calm and alert, reported no allergies and was not taking any medication. He had no past history of significant medical problems and had eaten dinner four hours ago, which included a six-pack of beer. There was no other recent trauma or illness.

O: The patient was awake but subdued, with normal mental status. He had two small puncture wounds on his left forearm. There was minimal swelling extending 7 centimeters proximal to the bite, but no discoloration. The area was mildly tender to the touch. Distal CSM was intact. There were no other injuries. Vital signs at 1015 were BP: unavailable, P: 80, R: 16, T: appears normal, Skin: W/D/P, C: Awake and oriented.

A: 1. Pit viper bite.

2. Dark, windy conditions

A': 1. Local and systemic effects of toxin.

2. Hazardous evacuation.

P: Vital signs and CSM checks were done every fifteen minutes. No progress of symptoms was noted over the next three hours. The patient was monitored overnight and evacuated by boat in the morning. A complete SOAP note was written and sent with the patient.

Discussion: The decision to stay in camp was based on the low risk of further serious problems from the snakebite, and the high risk of waterborne evacuation in the dark. Proceeding with evacuation in the morning was appropriate, even though symptoms had not progressed. Problems with blood coagulation and compartment syndrome can develop later and should be monitored. ✚

Chapter 12

Thermoregulation

The core of the human body operates most efficiently at or very near a temperature of 37 degrees C. The brain adjusts heat production and retention automatically based on information from temperature sensors in the skin and body core. Blood vessels in the skin dilate or constrict to dissipate or preserve heat. Sweat glands release fluid to enhance cooling by evaporation. Shivering produces heat with involuntary exercise. You can watch these compensation mechanisms at work, but they are not under your direct control.

Our conscious efforts are also an important factor affecting the ability of our thermoregulatory system to compensate. You put on or shed clothing, seek the shade when you're hot, or lie in sun like a lizard when you're cold. You curl up to preserve heat, or spread yourself out to get rid of it. Your intelligence and freedom of movement are important factors in striking the balance. Unfortunately, problems with heat and cold often have their origins in poor judgment.

Problems with thermoregulation can also develop when the function of the thermoregulatory system becomes impaired by illness, injury, toxins, or medication. The system can also be overwhelmed by environmental extremes. Subsequent changes in body core temperature, fluid volume, and energy stores further impair the system. The patient is doomed without aggressive intervention. Maintaining or correcting the function of the thermoregulatory system is a key element of patient care in the wilderness setting.

Compensation Factors

Voluntary Efforts:

• Clothing and shelter

• Eating and drinking

Fitness and morphology:

• Larger muscle mass generates more heat.

• Long and thin people lose heat more quickly.

• Fit people generate heat more easily.

• Acclimatized people dissipate heat more easily.

Hypothermia

Our good friend and colleague, John Haskins, was a superb Outward Bound instructor. He's had a lot of firsthand experience with hypothermia. John has spent way too much time in small, open boats off the coast of Maine.

No one could design a better laboratory for studying the effects of long-term exposure to cold and wet environments. One of the first things to be affected by hypothermia is judgment and common sense. The fact that John kept teaching for so many years seems to prove this point.

The Maine coast is particularly good at inducing hypothermia: a low ambient temperature; wetness in the form of rain, fog, and general high humidity; and wind. To counter the challenge, John used passive heat retention in the form of insulation (fat and winter clothing), and constriction of the blood vessels in the skin to keep warmth in the body core. He also reduced the area of his body exposed to heat loss by curling up in the bottom of the boat. By this time John was usually cold, shivering, and miserable.

He was quick to recognize the cold response and his body's attempt to produce heat. He would usually leap to an oar and row briskly to help with active heat production. His students thought he was crazy, but John always began to feel better. He also knew that in order to produce heat, he needed calories to burn. This was a perfect excuse to eat something. Then John felt much better. He was still at sea and lost in the fog, but at least he was warm.

COLD RESPONSE

Cold response is a normal reaction to feeling cold and begins long before the body core temperature begins to fall with the onset of hypothermia. Shell/core compensation reduces heat loss to the environment while shivering increases heat production from muscle activity. The discomfort you feel by being cold motivates your conscious effort to add layers of clothing and get out of the weather. If the system works normally and is not overwhelmed by an extreme challenge, normal core temperature and mental status are preserved.

Nobody will be able to mount an effective cold response when short on food and fluids. Shivering is a very efficient form of heat production but requires a tremendous amount of energy. Living outside in a cold environment can require more than 6,000 calories a day. Normal body fluid volume is also required to effectively generate and distribute heat.

An anticipated and annoying problem associated with the cold response is "cold diuresis." This is the tendency of the body to produce more urine as blood is shunted from the shell into the core. Cold diuresis and the logistics involved in obtaining fresh water in an extreme environment can lead to dehydration.

Although cold response is normal and healthy, it carries the anticipated problem of hypothermia. A number of factors can accelerate the process. A patient who is immobilized by injury will not be able to exercise or protect themselves from heat loss. Drugs that cause vasodilation of the skin will result in greater heat loss. Chronic disease states can inhibit the body's ability to sense or respond to temperature changes, preventing adequate heat production and distribution. Elderly people have less muscle mass and a reduced ability to perceive and respond to heat loss. Children tend to have less body fat and a greater surface area to mass ratio, which will also increase the rate of heat loss.

Reversing cold response requires insulation, protection, calories, and fluids. To do this most effectively, you will need to understand the physics of heat production, retention, and dissipation. Heat energy is transferred from warmer objects, like your body, to colder objects, like the ground. The mechanisms are *conduction, convection, evaporation,* and *radiation.*

Conduction is heat transfer between objects in contact. The more dense the object, the faster heat energy will be transferred. You will lose heat much more quickly to the cold, hard ground than to the low-density foam pad that you should be sitting on. Water will conduct heat from the body about twenty-five times faster than air.

Convection is heat transfer via moving fluids, including air and water. Although air is the least dense substance, there is an infinite supply of it. Heat lost to wind, or even the air billowing in and out of loose clothing, can be considerable. Water works the same way, just many times faster.

Evaporation refers to the heat energy absorbed by water as it turns into water vapor. The body uses this very efficient mechanism for cooling in the form of sweat. Water evaporating from the skin will cool you very efficiently whether you need it or not.

Radiant heat energy is emitted and absorbed by all objects, including your body. This energy is the warmth you feel from sunlight or a campfire. Radiant heat from your body can be absorbed and reflected back to you by dense clothing or a reflective foil covering. This is how some insulation can be so effective while remaining so thin.

In protecting yourself in a cold environment, you must consider all forms of heat loss. Noncompressible insulation, such as a closed-cell foam pad, will reduce conductive heat loss to the ground or other cold objects. High-loft, low-density insulation, such as a synthetic or down sleeping bag, reduces convective heat loss and traps the radiant heat being emitted by your body. Keeping yourself dry reduces evaporative cooling.

Support for heat production is equally critical. You will need calories and fluids to fuel shivering. Simple sugars are best at first. They will be quickly absorbed and converted into energy. Complex carbohydrates, fats, and protein can be added later to maintain heat production.

Adding heat in the form of warm liquids or heat packs to a cold person is comforting but not as useful as calories, hydration, and exercise. The heat energy in a cup of hot tea is minimal compared to the heat that will be produced when your cold hiking partner burns the four tablespoons of honey you put into it. Don't delay food and fluids while waiting for your stove to heat up.

Most of the time, your efforts will be successful. Sometimes, the system fails or is overwhelmed by environmental conditions, resulting in a drop in body core temperature. Shell/core compensation persists, shivering continues, and your partner's mental status begins to decay. Your anticipated problem has become the existing problem.

MILD HYPOTHERMIA

Any idiot can diagnose hypothermia in someone who's been overboard in the Gulf of Maine for forty minutes. The usual case, however, creeps up on you because you allow yourself or someone else to be just a little cold for a long time. In most backcountry situations the onset of hypothermia is more likely to be insidious than dramatic.

Hypothermia may be the primary problem you are treating or a side effect of environmental conditions. It is a common complication in trauma cases where an injured person has remained immobile for hours while waiting for rescue. It also develops in rescue team members waiting for hours for something to happen.

In rapid-onset cases like cold-water immersion, there is often a radical difference in temperature between the cold body shell and the still relatively warm body core. Generally, the patient has not had time to become significantly dehydrated or calorie depleted. This is called *acute hypothermia,* and spontaneous rewarming is usually possible once the patient has been removed from the water, dried, and insulated.

In slow-onset cases, called *subacute hypothermia,* glycogen stores and blood sugar are often depleted. The patient is usually dehydrated. The temperature difference between shell and core is not as dramatic. These patients will not be able to rewarm without help. In fact, rewarming efforts can be lethal without hydration and food.

Mild Hypothermia

Mechanism:

- Heat loss exceeds heat production.
- Onset can be acute or subacute.

Signs and Symptoms:

- Mild to moderate mental status changes
- Shivering
- Shell/core effect
- Body core temperature 35 - 32°C

Mild Hypothermia

Treatment:

- Immediate field rewarming
- Food and fluids
- Trap heat generated by shivering
- Insulate from convection, conduction, radiation
- Dry skin and clothing to reduce evaporation
- Exercise only when improvement is noted
- Package and evacuate if not improving

The most obvious signs of mild hypothermia are mental status changes and shivering. The patient may be lethargic, withdrawn, confused, or exhibit personality changes. A normally pleasant crew member may become irritable and hostile. A person who is normally loud and unpleasant may become quiet and complacent (which is particularly dangerous because there will be tremendous temptation to leave him that way). Body core temperature will measure below 35 degrees C. Shivering can be mild to severe. If the patient is not already dehydrated, cold diuresis will continue with the patient producing relatively dilute urine.

The most accurate body core temperature measurements are made by esophageal probe, not usually available in your local hardware store. Rectal measurements would be the next most accurate. A special low reading clinical thermometer is required for measuring core temperature below 34 degrees C.

As a general rule, any patient who can vigorously protest the use of a rectal thermometer is not significantly hypothermic. In any case the measurement of core temperature is not necessary to make the diagnosis. Any cold person with altered mental status is hypothermic.

Treatment of Mild Hypothermia: Mild hypothermia is an urgent problem requiring immediate and aggressive treatment in the field. The anticipated problem, severe hypothermia, will be much more difficult to handle. The treatment is essentially the same as that for cold response: protect from heat loss and restore calories and fluid.

Vigorous shivering is the most efficient form of field rewarming for the mildly hypothermic person. It just needs fluid and fuel. Adding external heat with hot water bottles or a campfire is generally safe and certainly more comfortable, but no attempt to exercise the person should be made until obvious improvement in mental status is noted, especially in subacute hypothermia.

All hypothermic people experience some degree of afterdrop, where the body core temperature continues to decrease even after rewarming has begun. This is due to the physics of heat transfer through any medium, but is accentuated by dilation of the skin blood vessels and circulation of the blood through the cooler extremities as the person rewarms. As a result, your partner may get a little worse before getting better, especially if you exercise him too soon. It may require more than forty minutes of shivering, sugar, fluids, and aggressive external rewarming before it becomes safe to allow him to exercise.

SEVERE HYPOTHERMIA

For hospital treatment, several distinct stages of hypothermia are defined to guide the resuscitation effort. Most commonly these are referred to as mild, moderate, and severe. For field treatment, however, the distinction is mostly practical: Can the patient cooperate with your treatment or not? A very cold person who is not awake, cannot move about on his own, is not shivering, and cannot protect his own airway is treated as severely hypothermic. An accurate measurement of core temperature is not required.

As the core temperature falls below 32 degrees C, mental status changes will become severe, followed by a drop to V, P, or U on the AVPU scale. This is quite different from the subdued but awake mild hypothermic. Shivering will stop as muscles are deactivated by shell cooling and lack of calories to burn. Cold diuresis may continue if fluid stores are not yet depleted.

Severe Hypothermia

Signs and Symptoms:

- V, P, or U on AVPU
- Shell/core effect
- No shivering
- Core temperature < 32°C

Complications:

- Cardiac irritability
- Dehydration, metabolic derangement
- VS may be undetectable

Treatment of Severe Hypothermia: The ideal treatment for severe hypothermia is controlled rewarming in a hospital, preferably a level one trauma center. Package the patient to prevent heat loss before initiating a gentle but urgent evacuation.

The package should include heat sources such as warm water bottles or a charcoal heat pack applied to the chest area. Positive pressure ventilation with heated air may also help. This will minimize heat loss and may actually begin the rewarming process. Because rough handling can cause the cold heart to go into ventricular fibrillation, keep the patient horizontal and transport as gently as you can.

Severe Hypothermia

Field Treatment and Evacuation:

- Package with added heat source to begin rewarming
- Urgent but gentle evacuation to hospital maintained in horizontal position
- PPV with heated and humidified oxygen
- Warmed IV if available
- No chest compressions

"Avoid aggressive external rewarming, like immersion in a hot tub… because this may induce peripheral vasodilatation and shock."

In extremely cold patients, pulse and respiration may not be detectable. It is quite possible to mistake severe hypothermia for death. Anecdotal experience and animal studies suggest that even people in apparent cardiac arrest may be treatable if the body core temperature is above 10 degrees C and you can get the person to a hospital within three hours. Your thermometer can help make the distinction between a patient and a body recovery.

Field rewarming of the severe hypothermic should be considered a last resort to be applied if timely evacuation would be dangerous or impossible. Find shelter and apply heat any way that you can, but try to avoid aggressive external rewarming like immersion in a hot spring or exposure to a hot engine room because this may induce peripheral vasodilation and shock. Add sugar orally if the patient rewarms enough to protect his airway. If you succeed, recognize that metabolic derangement may be significant, and evacuation to medical care is still the ideal when it can be accomplished.

If your patient is in apparent cardiac arrest and you are more than three hours from a hospital, try to warm him enough to produce detectable vital signs. If no pulse or other life signs are observed after thirty minutes of external heat and PPV, the effort should be discontinued. You have given it a try, but there is no chance of success.

▶ Case Study #1: Hypothermia

S: A seventeen-year-old student was removed from the bow of a pulling boat after being on watch without relief for three hours during a cold and wet sail to windward. He had repeatedly been asked if he was cold, or would like something to eat, and always replied, "okay." He responded the same way when asked if he saw anything ahead. Because no one else was particularly excited about replacing him, he remained at his post. Eventually, someone noticed that his wool hat had rolled down over his eyes even though he continued to claim to be on lookout. After some debate among the students, this was brought to the instructor's attention.

The student had no known allergies, he was not on medication, he had no history of significant medical problems, and his last meal was more than four hours before. There was no reason to suspect injury.

O: On examination, the student was awake but subdued and confused. He could open his eyes and sit up on command. His foul weather gear was open in front and he was soaked to the waist. Vital signs at 1615 were BP: 110/70, P: 60, R: 12, C: A on AVPU with lethargy and confusion, T: felt cool, Skin: pale.

A: Mild hypothermia

A': Severe hypothermia

P: Sail was reduced and the boat was turned downwind. One student was detailed to start the stove, and another to replace the patient on watch. Other students removed the patient's soaked gear. He was clothed in borrowed polypropylene, placed in a doubled sleeping bag, and wrapped in a plastic tarp. He was assisted in drinking a couple of cups of warm, thick cocoa.

Discussion: Although this problem could have been avoided, it was handled appropriately once discovered. The instructor's plan stabilized

---

Severe Hypothermia
Wilderness Context

<u>No Chance of Survival:</u>

- Obvious lethal injury
- The chest is frozen
- The core temperature is below 10°C
- Submerged underwater more than one hour

---

the scene, reduced the cold challenge, and increased heat retention and production.

This fellow showed almost immediate improvement in consciousness and mental status. Evacuation was not initiated, but the instructor chose to continue downwind to an anchorage several miles away. The expedition was continued in the same messy and cold easterly wind the following day, but the entire crew was warm, well fed, and hydrated. Bow watch was rotated regularly.

Heat-Related Illness

Sources of heat energy are both internal and external. Inside your body heat is constantly being produced as a by-product of metabolism and increases dramatically with exercise. Because your vital organs work best at a temperature of around 37 degrees C, the body will conserve only as much heat as it needs to keep it there and will get rid of the rest. Your primary tool for dumping excess heat is the dilation of blood vessels in your skin and the evaporation of sweat. The body constantly sacrifices fluid to maintain normal temperature in hot environments.

When the blood vessels in the skin are fully dilated, they can contain as much as 3,000 milliliters of warm blood. In order for the water in sweat to evaporate, it has to absorb a tremendous amount of heat energy from the blood near the skin surface. This is a very effective cooling system as long as there is enough blood and sweat to keep it going.

You might remember your junior high science teacher telling you that it takes one calorie of heat energy to raise one gram of water one degree Celsius. That's merely interesting. But consider that it takes 540 calories to evaporate one gram of water into water vapor. That's important. Now you know why sweating can cool you so well, and why you had to memorize this in seventh-grade science.

External sources of heat energy include not only warm air in the surrounding environment or inside your clothes but also the humidity of the air and your exposure to wind. This directly affects the efficiency of the heat loss mechanism. Moving air speeds evaporation and the conduction of heat away from the body, and dry air allows faster evaporation than humid air.

Like cold response, heat response is a normal process. As long as heat dissipation can keep up with heat production, the body core temperature will remain normal. Heat response should be treated with fluid replacement and reduction in heat exposure and production. In the backcountry setting, heat response carries the anticipated problems of heat exhaustion and heat stroke.

Heat exhaustion is primarily a body fluid volume problem caused by sweating. Body temperature may be mildly elevated, but that is not yet the main concern. Heat stroke is primarily a body core temperature problem caused by too much heat. The patient may also be dehydrated, but it is the elevated temperature that is the biggest threat. Another illness called hyponatremia may develop as a result of prevention and treatment. This problem is created by diluting the amount of salt in the blood and body tissues.

HEAT EXHAUSTION

This is the beginning of trouble. Heat exhaustion is actually early volume shock caused by dehydration due to sweating. Sweat can evaporate so quickly in dry climates that profuse sweating may go unnoticed until fluid loss is severe. Pay special attention to fluid replacement when the signs of heat response are present. Reduced urine output is a good indicator that the body is compensating for reduced fluid intake or increased losses.

Body core temperature may be mildly elevated, but the primary problem is fluid depletion. You will recognize the vital sign pattern as mild compensated volume shock, including the shell/core effect. In the backcountry, heat exhaustion is a serious problem that requires immediate treatment.

Heat Exhaustion

Signs and Symptoms:

- Awake, normal mental status
- Sweating, near normal core temperature
- Vital sign pattern for volume shock

Treatment:

- Reduce exercise and heat exposure
- IV or PO fluids and food
- Evacuate if unable to rehydrate

Treatment of Heat Exhaustion: Reduce heat by moving the patient into the shade. Stop physical exertion, fan the patient with air, and assist evaporative cooling with water sprinkled on the skin. The object is to stop the progression of volume shock by preventing further dehydration through sweating. Radical cooling, such as immersion in ice water, is not necessary.

Fluid replacement should begin immediately. Oral intake is adequate, but intravenous fluid replacement is faster if that service is available. Oral replacement is still possible even if the patient is vomiting by giving fluid frequently in small amounts. Look for normal urine production and normal mental status as an indication of the return of normal fluid volume. Without IV fluids it may take more than twelve hours to bring the dehydrated person back to normal.

Replacing salt is also a good idea following heavy sweating. Salt, if you're worried about it, is provided by most foods and sports drinks. Do not give salt tablets, which cause stomach irritation and vomiting.

HEAT STROKE

This is a life-threatening emergency requiring immediate field treatment. The person will probably be dehydrated, but the primary problem is dangerously elevated body core temperature capable of significant damage to the brain and vital organs. Symptoms include unmistakable changes in mental status and hot skin.

Sweating has usually stopped, but it is possible for a critical rise in core temperature to occur before the patient has time to become dehydrated. In these cases, the skin may be still wet with sweat. This extreme rise in core temperature can be caused by forced exercise in a hot environment, such as fighting a wildland fire, or from sitting too long in a very hot sauna.

Regardless of the fluid status or how quick the onset, these people look very sick. The key indicators are a positive mechanism for hyperthermia, a high core temperature, and any changes in mental status.

Heat Stroke

Mechanism:

- High heat challenge, environmental and/or metabolic
- Inadequate cooling

Signs and Symptoms:

- Profound mental status changes, seizures
- Hot, dry or sweating. Temp > 40°C
- Vital sign pattern for volume shock
- Skin may be red, or pale with shell/core

Treatment of Heat Stroke: There is no time for delay. Immediate cooling is required. Immersion in cold water will certainly work but is not always available. You can also spray the patient with water and fan her with air, taking advantage of evaporative cooling. Look for an improvement in level of consciousness and mental status to determine the return of more normal temperature. The ability to measure core temperature may be useful here. Beware that cold-water immersion can result in a rapid swing toward hypothermia.

Fluid replacement is critical but only after core temperature is being effectively treated. Intravenous fluid replacement is ideal, but oral fluids may work if the patient can cooperate and protect her airway.

Emergency evacuation is justified. These patients are best served by treatment and observation in the hospital. Brain swelling is possible, with the anticipated problem of increasing ICP. A condition called rhabdomyolysis may develop, leading to liver and kidney failure. Field care should include rest and aggressive oral hydration to maintain normal urine output.

Heat Stroke

Treatment:

- Stop exercise, remove from hot environment
- Immediate and radical cooling
- IV or PO fluids and electrolytes
- Evacuation after cooling is ideal
- Evacuation may be non-emergent if vital signs and mental status return to normal
- Long-term care should include hydration for normal urine output

Wilderness Context

High Risk Problem:

- VS do not return to normal
- Persistent altered mental status
- Decreased urine output
- Urine color becomes red or brown
- You cannot prevent exposure to heat
- The patient is getting worse

EXERTIONAL HYPONATREMIA

Exertional hyponatremia is caused by drinking too much water, sweating a lot, and not taking in enough salt. This is usually a problem for extreme athletes, wildland firefighters, and others who are acutely aware of the need to maintain hydration but don't take the time to eat enough. It is magnified in people who are not acclimatized to the heat, and thus losing excessive amounts of salt through sweat. The person dilutes the salt content of the body to a point where function is impaired. The term "hyponatremia" means low sodium, one of the body's primary electrolytes.

The signs and symptoms can resemble heat exhaustion with weakness, nausea, and headache. But hyponatremia typically causes changes in mental status, including slow thinking and confusion. Another essential difference is near-normal urine volume. The urine will also be relatively dilute.

Exertional Hyponatremia

Mechanism:

- Loss of fluid and electrolytes through sweat
- Inadequate electrolyte replacement

Signs and Symptoms:

- Altered mental status, slow mentation, tremors, seizures
- Nausea, headache, weakness
- Near normal urine output
- Core temperature normal

Treatment:

- Salty food
- Rest
- Restore fluid volume
- Evacuate if not improving

"Sometimes improvement is immediate with the ingestion of salty foods."

Treatment of Exertional Hyponatremia: Water restriction and electrolyte replacement are the usual treatment. Sometimes improvement is immediate with the ingestion of salty foods. If there is evidence that the person is also dehydrated, volume replacement may also be necessary. As with any problem, if the patient is not improving quickly or getting worse, evacuation to medical care is indicated. ✚

Chapter 13
Cold Injury

The expansion of water as it turns to ice is an impressive natural force. Frost action crumbles mountain ranges, cracks engine blocks, and heaves roads. When freezing occurs in your fingers and toes, the effects are no less impressive.

Anything that restricts the circulation of warm blood to tissues allows freezing to occur more readily. In people who are already a little chilled, the shell/core effect reduces perfusion to the extremities to maintain core temperature. Tight clothing such as ski boots or a splint tied too tightly can reduce blood flow as well. Cigarette smoking is an additional factor, infusing the body tissues with nicotine, which is a powerful vasoconstrictor.

I will forever be amazed by the sight of a lightly dressed skier huddled on the chairlift with the temperature below zero, having his morning cigarette. He should just take off all of his clothes, jump in the snow, and get it over with! Few of them seem to see what skiing hatless and smoking has to do with frostbitten toes. The ski boots are usually blamed.

This is not such a big deal at a ski resort with lodges top and bottom. But in the backcountry dealing with frostbite is inconvenient at best and often disastrous. It must be taken seriously both in prevention and in cure.

Certainly, well-insulated and fitted boots, gloves, and a face mask can go a long way toward preventing frostbite in extreme conditions. But equally important is maintaining an active and warm body core. This will ensure a good supply of warm blood to the extremities. That's why you eat a good breakfast and wear a hat to keep your feet warm.

Frostbite

Sometime when you're not paying attention or are a little hypothermic and not thinking clearly enough to prevent it, tissues will begin to freeze. You won't feel it happening. Because nerve tissue is the most sensitive to oxygen deprivation, the affected part goes numb when the circulation stops. Ice crystals form, doing the same kind of damage ice can do anywhere.

Severe damage can result with prolonged or very deep freezing. Much of the damage occurs during and after rewarming. Rewarmed tissue is very sensitive to further injury, even from normal use. Refreezing is devastating. For a good example of the potential for damage, freeze and thaw a ripe tomato a couple of times. You'll be left with a pile of red mush.

The very early stage of freezing is called "frostnip." This occurs when there is a loss of local tissue perfusion with the beginning of ice crystal formation. Only the outer layers of skin are affected, and damage is minimal. The area will appear white or gray in Caucasian people and pink or red in dark-skinned people and feel cold and stiff to the touch. However, the area will remain pliable enough to allow movement over unfrozen deeper skin layers, joints, and tendons. The typical discomfort of early cooling will be replaced by numbness. Prompt rewarming at this stage usually causes no disability or tissue loss.

Frostnip responds rapidly to rewarming with minimal pain and only mild inflammation following. The rewarmed skin will be mildly tender, red, and slightly swollen. Blistering does not occur. No specific long-term care is required, although the skin will be more susceptible to further cold injury.

Frostbite occurs when the skin and underlying tissues are frozen solid. The area is white or bluish and firm to touch. Skin does not move over joints or underlying tissues. Ice crystals are usually visible on the skin surface. There is a complete loss of sensation. The digit or extremity feels like a club.

Rewarming is extremely painful and can cause further damage if not done properly. The rewarmed tissues do not look or feel normal. There will be signs of mild to severe inflammation with blisters, swelling, and redness. There may be some death of tissue, which will appear dark blue or black.

Frostbite

Assessment:

- Superficial
  - Soft, pale or red, painful to dulled sensation
  - Also called *frostnip*
- Partial Thickness
  - Soft, pale, cold, numb
  - Involves dermis only
  - Moves freely over subcutaneous tissue
- Full Thickness
  - Hard, pale or blue, no sensation
  - Frozen into subcutaneous tissue
  - Involved joints do not move

Treatment of Frostbite: Frostnip should be immediately rewarmed at the first sign of numbness. Left frozen, frostnip can easily progress to frostbite. Like early hypothermia, frostnip is a case for stopping whatever you're doing and making the time and effort to warm up. Any method that does not cause tissue damage is fine. Usually, just protecting the area from the weather will do it. Remember to warm the whole body as well as the affected part. Reverse the shell/core effect. Put a hat on, eat something, and exercise to produce heat. The people who get into trouble with frostbite are the ones who ignore the first signs of frostnip.

Frostbite is best treated by rewarming under controlled conditions. The chances of further damage from trauma and infection are high. Pain will be severe. Usually this means the patient should be in a medical facility. Allowing tissue to remain frozen for several hours during an evacuation is better than uncontrolled field rewarming. This is especially true of frozen feet and hands, which will be impossible to use once rewarmed (remember the tomato).

Frostbite

Treatment:

- **Superficial and Partial Thickness**
  - Immediate field rewarming
  - Reverse shell/core effect
  - Protect from refreezing
- **Full Thickness**
  - Ideal: controlled rewarming in the hospital
  - Pre-treat with ibuprofen 800 mg p.o.
  - Consider narcotics for additional pain control
  - Immerse in 37 – 40.5° C water until warm

If you find yourself stuck somewhere that makes evacuation impossible to accomplish within twenty-four hours or so, field rewarming may be your only option. Set up a secure shelter and be sure your patient is warm, dry, well fed, and hydrated. Premedicate with an anti-inflammatory drug such as ibuprofen (800 milligrams) taken by mouth. This will reduce pain and inflammation and help prevent blood clots in the injured tissue. Immerse the frozen extremity in warm water water between 37 and 40.5 degrees C. If you don't have a thermometer, the water should feel hot, but not uncomfortable, to normal skin. Keep adding warm water to the pot to keep the temperature up as the thawing process continues.

Once the part is rewarmed, it is vital to protect it from trauma. This means no use of the digit or extremity. Absolutely never allow the part to refreeze.

Consider rewarmed frostbite to be a high-risk wound. Bandages and splinting are required. Rewarmed frostbite on the feet usually means a helicopter or carry-out evacuation when that becomes possible.

Monitor distal circulation, sensation, and movement frequently to ensure that splints or bandages do not constrict circulation as swelling develops. If possible, keep the part elevated. Continue regular doses of ibuprofen. If you have it, cover the area with aloe vera gel or ointment, which has been shown to have both anti-inflammatory and antibacterial properties. Early medical follow-up is essential.

Frostbite that rewarms spontaneously during an evacuation should be protected the same way. Do not try to prevent rewarming by packing an extremity in snow. If it starts to thaw, stop where you are and deal with it.

Full Thickness Frostbite
Wilderness Context

Field Treatment if:

- Evacuation will exceed 24 hours
- Use of the extremity will not be necessary for survival and evacuation
- Re-freezing can be prevented
- The equipment is available

"Once the part is rewarmed, it is vital to protect it from trauma…Absolutely never allow the part to refreeze."

Trench Foot

Trench foot is an injury that develops with prolonged exposure to cold and wet conditions above freezing. It is not limited to feet and often involves the hands of paddlers, anglers, and others working or playing on the water. The injury is a result of prolonged vasoconstriction and tissue breakdown, an example of ischemia to infarction.

Trench Foot

Mechanism:

- Prolonged cold exposure, > 0° C
- Vasoconstriction and loss of local perfusion
- Ischemia to Infarction in skin tissue
- Inflammation and secondary infection

Treatment:

- Dry and warm
- Preserve perfusion, reverse shell/core
- Clean, treat infection as necessary
- NSAIDs

With the death of some of the tissue cells, inflammation develops, causing redness, pain, and swelling. Blisters can occur, with the possibility of secondary infection where the dermis has been exposed. Walking may become difficult or impossible.

Treatment of Trench Foot (or hand): If the cause is wet and cold, common sense would suggest that the treatment is warm and dry. Like frostbite, healing tissue can be damaged by further use. Bandaging for protection may be required. Treat any open wounds to prevent infection and allow healing.

Prevention is worth the trouble. In "trench" conditions try to give your hands and feet several dry and warm hours each day. Sleep with your wet socks in your sleeping bag to dry, but not with them on your feet. Take your wet suit booties and gloves off whenever possible. Inside waterproof boots, change your socks frequently to keep your feet as dry as you can. ✚

Chapter 14

Submersion Injury

Drowning is death by respiratory failure because some liquid replaces the air in the lung. The liquid is usually water and generally gets in when the patient inhales part of the lake, ocean, or river in which he or she is submerged.

The most common cause of drowning is loss of muscular coordination due to the rapid shell cooling that occurs in cold-water immersion. No longer able to swim, the victim sinks below the surface and inhales water. Even the strongest swimmer can drown this way.

Drowning can also happen almost instantly with the involuntary gasp that sometimes comes with the surprise of sudden immersion. This can affect kayakers rolled by a wave, or anglers pulled out of the boat by their pot warp or nets. They are immediately deprived of any reserve air and will not remain conscious for more than a few seconds. Most of the time, water fills the lungs all the way to the alveoli. In about 15 percent of the cases, the larynx goes into spasm, closing off the lungs, resulting in a "dry drowning." In either case, a water-filled respiratory system is unhealthy but not always fatal.

The term "submersion injury" describes the problems experienced by people who survive prolonged immersion in water without drowning. The most profound issue is brain damage from hypoxia. Another significant complication is the development of pulmonary edema due to irritation of lung tissue by inhaled water.

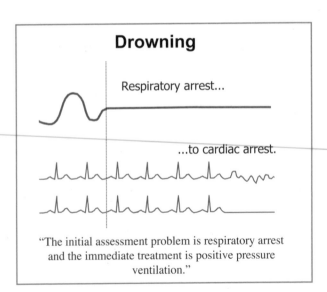

Drowning

Respiratory arrest...

...to cardiac arrest.

"The initial assessment problem is respiratory arrest and the immediate treatment is positive pressure ventilation."

Most people who survive submersion rescue themselves. Such an event with no loss of consciousness and no persistent respiratory symptoms indicates that hypoxia was not significant and water inhalation did not occur. This person may be uncomfortable and scared but is not at risk for developing critical system problems as a result of submersion. It is the victim who has lost consciousness or had to be rescued and resuscitated who will have inhaled water and be at risk for later complications.

You may have heard about people surviving submersion of an hour or more. This occurs in very cold water where the rapid cooling of the brain offers temporary protection from the damage caused by the lack of oxygen. In rare cases in the civilized setting, patients have been resuscitated after up to an hour under cold water. What is meant by "cold" is controversial. Generally, though, any water below about 20 degrees C can be considered cold enough to have the desired effect. The degree of protection offered by the onset of hypothermia increases considerably as water temperature goes down.

Treatment of Submersion Injury: Most of the people who survive submersion were not deprived of oxygen long enough to cause cardiac arrest. With prompt PPV they usually begin breathing on their own within a couple of minutes. Even though they may appear to be much better immediately after rescue, they should be quickly evacuated to medical care. Water is an irritant to lung tissue and will cause the later development of pulmonary edema. In effect, the patient will begin to drown again as the lungs fill up with water from inside the body.

Respiratory Arrest

Treatment:
- PPV as needed
- Hypothermia package
- Evacuate, anticipate:
  - hypothermia
  - pulmonary edema
  - increased ICP

"It is the patient who has lost consciousness or had to be rescued and resuscitated whom you should worry about."

People who are submerged for long enough to suffer cardiac arrest are much less likely to survive resuscitation in the field. Nevertheless, if it will not endanger rescuers, resuscitation should be attempted if the victim has been under water for less than an hour. The best chance for survival occurs with young patients submerged in near-freezing fresh water in close proximity to sophisticated medical care. Respiratory failure is treated immediately with positive pressure ventilation. Confirmed cardiac arrest is treated with CPR. There is no need to drain water from the lungs, and there is no difference in field treatment between salt and fresh water.

People who are successfully resuscitated from cardiac arrest are at risk for pulmonary edema from water inhalation and increasing ICP from brain damage due to hypoxia. Patients who do not respond quickly to basic life support do not survive. Resuscitation efforts beyond the thirty-minute CPR protocols are not justified. ✚

Cardiac Arrest

Treatment:
- Attempt resuscitation with CPR if submersion is less than one hour
- Urban – immediate ALS and hospital transfer
- Wilderness – follow CPR protocols

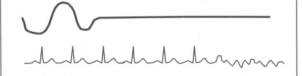

Chapter 15
Altitude Illness

The higher you go, the less oxygen there is. At about 18,000 feet above sea level, air pressure (hence, air available to breathe) is reduced by 50 percent. This is accentuated at higher latitude because the earth's atmosphere is thicker at the equator and thinner at the poles. For example, the effects of altitude on the summit of Denali in Alaska are about 15 percent greater than at the same altitude in the Himalayas.

At a constant altitude, the amount of oxygen in the air is constant. It does not fluctuate significantly with the temperature, time of day, season, or any other routine environmental changes. Your critical body systems become accustomed to this. Your rate of respiration, the number of red blood cells in your circulation, and other physiologic parameters are in balance with your environment, whether you're a Maine lobsterman or a mountain guide in the Andes.

There are compensatory mechanisms that allow you to change altitude, within limits, without getting out of balance. You can move from sea level to about 2,500 meters with minimal effect. In the short term there will be an increase in respiratory rate to make up for the reduced oxygen. Because you are breathing faster, you will blow off more CO_2 than usual, causing your blood to become more basic (elevated pH). If you stay at altitude several days, your kidneys will rebalance the pH of the blood, resetting your system to your new environment.

Compensation for Altitude

Short Term:

- Hyperventilation
- Tachycardia and increased blood pressure

Long Term:

- Body produces more red blood cells and hemoglobin
- Capillary beds increase in density

If you were to continue even higher, your body would compensate and rebalance again. Over the course of weeks you would undergo further physiologic changes, such as producing more red blood cells. Ultimately, you would reach the limit of your body's ability to compensate.

This ability of your body to adapt to altitude, and the speed with which it happens, varies widely from person to person. Women seem to be less susceptible to respiratory problems, but otherwise there appears to be no relationship to physical fitness or gender. Some people adapt to altitude better than others. However, everyone's ability to adapt to higher altitudes is reduced by alcohol and other depressant drugs, which reduce the nervous system's respiratory drive. Overexertion at the new altitude also inhibits acclimatization.

The best way to adapt to higher altitude is to take your time, stay away from depressants, and take it easy. Allow your normal compensatory mechanisms the time to work by ascending in stages. Climb no faster than your body can adapt. Do not overexert on the first day at the new altitude, and plan to remain for two or three days before proceeding higher. If you pay attention to what your body is trying to tell you, you should be able to avoid more serious problems.

Severe problems develop when the reduced oxygenation results in capillary leakage and body tissue swelling. The organs most seriously affected by this are the brain and lungs, resulting in the medical conditions we call high-altitude pulmonary edema (HAPE) and high-altitude cerebral edema (HACE). The generic problems, of course, are the familiar elevated intracranial pressure (ICP) and pulmonary fluid.

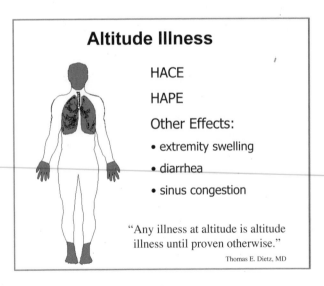

Altitude Illness

HACE

HAPE

Other Effects:

• extremity swelling

• diarrhea

• sinus congestion

"Any illness at altitude is altitude illness until proven otherwise."

Thomas E. Dietz, MD

Acute Mountain Sickness and HACE

A significant percentage of people who travel to altitudes above 2,500 meters experience some degree of acute mountain sickness. When the brain swelling progresses far enough to significantly increase ICP, the more serious symptoms of HACE appear. The exact mechanism for this capillary leakage of fluid into the brain is still largely unknown.

Mild acute mountain sickness is characterized by mild headache easily relieved by aspirin or ibuprofen and slight nausea with little or no vomiting. The patient may experience slight dizziness, loss of appetite, mild fatigue, and some degree of insomnia. This is where two days of prevention is worth 1,000 meters of cure.

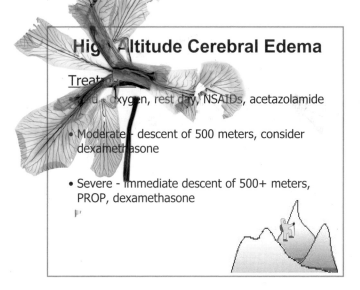

High Altitude Cerebral Edema

Treatment

oxygen, rest day, NSAIDs, acetazolamide

• Moderate - descent of 500 meters, consider dexamethasone

• Severe - immediate descent of 500+ meters, PROP, dexamethasone

Moderate HACE produces severe headaches not relieved by aspirin or ibuprofen, persistent vomiting, and fatigue. Theses are the typical symptoms of increased ICP, similar to what you might see following a traumatic brain injury. The patient is now at risk for dehydration and airway obstruction along with the possibility of continued brain swelling.

Severe HACE is a life-threatening emergency. Fortunately, it is rarely seen below 4,000 meters. The key feature is ataxia (inability to walk straight). The patient will show significant changes in mental status. The symptoms of severe HACE can be confused or mixed with those of other problems such as low blood sugar, dehydration, hypothermia, hyperthermia, and exercise exhaustion. All of these problems can cause a decrease in muscular performance and efficiency. All can cause changes in level of consciousness and mental status. Under most field conditions, the most practical approach is to include all five problems as possible causes until proven otherwise.

Prevention and Treatment of HACE: The key to prevention is to recognize acute mountain sickness, the mild form of HACE, and allow your body time to adapt before climbing any higher. You should avoid sedatives such as alcohol or narcotic drugs, which can depress respiration, but should use ibuprofen or aspirin for pain relief. A drug called acetazolamide, available by prescription, can be used to help your kidneys adjust your blood pH. Taking 125 mg twice a day is usually sufficient (please consult a medical practitioner).

Moderate HACE is treated with pain medication, rest, avoiding sedatives, and an immediate descent of 500 meters, if possible. The patient should be observed closely for increasing severity of symptoms. Be prepared for an emergency descent if his condition worsens. Supplemental oxygen will be helpful. For a short time, steroid drugs can be used to reduce swelling. A therapeutic dose of Decadron is 8 mg to start and 4 mg every six hours (again, please consult a medical practitioner).

Severe HACE is treated using all the techniques covered under the mild and moderate forms, *plus* an immediate descent of 1,000 meters. Exertion should be minimized, but there should be no delay in descent.

A portable device called a Gamow bag can be used to temporarily increase the air pressure around the patient by about 2 pounds per square inch, simulating a descent of 2,000 meters. This may substantially improve the patient's condition to the point that he or she can be released from the bag and allowed to walk down before debilitating symptoms recur.

High Altitude Pulmonary Edema

<u>Treatment:</u>
- Mild HAPE - oxygen, rest day, hydration and food, acetazolamide

- Moderate HAPE - immediate descent of 500 meters, consider nifedipine

- Severe HAPE - PROP, immediate descent of 500+ meters, nifedipine

---

High-Altitude Pulmonary Edema

High-altitude pulmonary edema (HAPE) is caused by constriction of pulmonary arteries in response to reduced levels of oxygen, in combination with increased cardiac output (stronger heartbeat). The increased pressure forces fluid out of the capillaries and into the alveoli, obstructing air exchange.

In its early stages, symptoms may be limited to mild shortness of breath with exertion and an infrequent cough. The condition may go unnoticed as anything but the effects of dry air. Many people probably experience early HAPE and recover without incident, never realizing what happened.

In its moderate form, HAPE is usually mistaken for a respiratory infection. HAPE can even cause a low-grade fever. The patient is coughing frequently and is noticeably short of breath with any degree of exertion. Fluid in the lungs can be heard as crackles through a stethoscope or an ear to the patient's chest.

Severe HAPE will cause shortness of breath even at rest and may produce gurgling respirations and a frequent cough productive of white or pink sputum. The patient will be in significant respiratory distress and appear cyanotic (blue or pale). Severe HAPE is an immediate threat to life.

Altitude Illness Prevention

- Above 3000 meters, ascend 300 – 1000 meters per day
- Rest days every 1000 – 1500 meters in ascent
- Carry high, sleep low
- Avoid CNS depressants
- Stay hydrated and well fed
- Be alert to early symptoms
- Prophylactic medications

Prevention and Treatment of HAPE: The appearance of any degree of HAPE is a bad sign. The condition tends to progress from bad to worse. Descent to a lower elevation should be a priority. Unfortunately, exertion will make pulmonary edema worse due to increased cardiac output. There may be situations where it would be better to remain where you are rather than perform a strenuous evacuation, especially if it involves going over a mountain pass before lower elevation is gained. A Gamow bag may be lifesaving.

If symptoms are severe, PROP should be applied with an emphasis on oxygen if it is available. A descent of 500 meters should improve symptoms. Unlike HACE, severe HAPE is not unusual at moderate altitudes between 2,500 and 4,000 meters.

Acetazolamide seems to be useful only in the early stages of HAPE, but other medications including nifedipine, sildinafil, and tadalafil have been shown to be effective in reducing pulmonary edema. There is also some evidence that inhaled albuterol, the drug used for asthma, may also help. If you are guiding above 3,000 meters, a discussion with a medical practitioner about these drugs and the authorization to use them should be considered. ✚

Chapter 16
Lightning Injuries

In the heart of a thunderstorm thousands of feet above an air base in eastern Ontario, the friction between violent air currents and particles of water and ice created an enormous negative electrostatic charge. Leader strokes probed toward the positively charged earth and were met 100 meters above the ground by a streamer probing upward from an Air Force jet parked on the apron. The newly established pathway became the conductor for a massive discharge of electrical current in a dazzling display of the natural phenomenon we call "lightning." Traveling through a channel of ionized air only about an inch in diameter, the current generated 15 million volts at 20,000 amperes in only 1/1000 of a second. The shock wave created by the explosive expansion of heated air rolled into the late afternoon as the familiar sound we call "thunder." The three air crewmen hiding from the rain under the jet's wing never heard it. They became part of the lightning pathway in an all-too-common example of what we like to call "bad luck."

The most seriously injured was found 6 meters from the aircraft. The only thing left of his clothing was his boots and necktie, and his pulse and breathing had stopped. He had a small burn on his chest where his dog tags had been resting. Only quick action by a St. John ambulance crew saved the man's life. Even though lightning can be capricious and unpredictable, there are some relatively safe places to shelter from a thunderstorm. Standing between a large metal object and the ground is not one of them.

Lightning is nature's way of equalizing the massive static electric charges that build up between the atmosphere and the ground during violent weather. The actual strike occurs when these charges build up enough potential to overcome atmospheric resistance. The trick is to avoid being there when it happens.

You know the obvious: Stay off hilltops and ridges, stay off the water, and generally try to avoid being the highest thing around. You also don't want to be in contact with an isolated tree, jet aircraft, or other likely target.

The height and isolation of an object are the only two factors that influence the likelihood of its being struck. In the field the best tactic is to squat or sit as low as you can, ideally on your foam pad or backpack, which will help insulate you from ground current. A group should be well spread out so that a strike will not incapacitate everybody at once. Aboard a larger boat, avoid having the whole crew clustered in the cockpit. Water is a good conductor, so don't swim or wade during a thunderstorm.

A relatively safe place is inside a car. The insulating value of the tires offers protection from ground current, and the metal shell will conduct the energy of a direct strike around the occupants and into the ground (likewise, our injured air crewman would have been much better off *inside* the aircraft). The metal shrouds and stays on a sailing vessel may have the same effect, provided there is a path to the water such as a good grounding system or heavy cable led over the side from a shroud. By the way, devices mounted on the masthead designed to "bleed off ions" or otherwise reduce the chances of a lightning strike do not work. In fact, if it increases the height of the rig, it will actually *increase* the risk of being struck.

Useful Information

- Isolation and height determine the likelihood of being struck
- Enclosed, grounded structures or vehicles are protective (surface effect)
- Ground current can travel up to 100 meters
- Current can jump gaps between conductors
- Metal and water can conduct current great distances
- Leader strokes travel about 30 – 50 meters

Lightning is second only to floods as the major weather killer in the United States and remains an occasional threat as far north as arctic Canada. You *do* have a better chance of being struck by lightning than buried in an avalanche, attacked by a shark, or sucked out of Kansas by a tornado.

The electrical discharge is well worth avoiding. It generates millions of volts and tens of thousands of amperes. You would think that this kind of power would utterly destroy anything in its path, but this is not always the case. Only about 10 percent of the people involved in a lightning strike die of their injuries.

In spite of its massive power, lightning is extremely brief in duration. The average discharge lasts for only about .001 second. This is not enough time for much of the electrical energy to overcome skin resistance and enter the body. Most of the current passes over the skin surface on its way to the ground. As a result, the types of internal injuries typical of household electrical current are rarely seen with lightning.

The current can affect you through direct contact if you're really unlucky, or indirectly in the form of ground current or splash-over. As the current passes through and over the tree you're leaning against, you can become part of the direct path. Splash-over can be best described as a much less powerful splinter of the main airborne bolt. Ground current spreads out through the earth, rock, or water from "ground zero." Because the energy is diffused, both forms of indirect exposure are generally less devastating than a direct hit.

The energy in lightning is dissipated in the form of heat and light. The instantaneous heating and expansion of the column of air through which the current passes generates the shock wave we hear as thunder. As with any explosion, if you are close enough, the shock wave can blow your eardrums, break bones, and rupture internal organs.

The direct current flow in a lightning strike can disrupt the electrochemical function of the nervous system, causing respiratory and cardiac arrest. As the current flows over the skin, it heats the moisture on the surface, causing superficial burns and, in some cases, enough explosive force to blow clothing apart.

Burns caused by lightning are generally superficial, with more serious deep burns occurring in less than 5 percent of patients. Nervous system disruption is common with many patients experiencing loss of consciousness, and most have some degree of memory loss. About 25 percent of survivors will develop significant long-term physical or psychological problems. The most common fatal event is cardiac and respiratory arrest.

The Scene Size-Up for dangers is particularly important in your response. Lightning does strike twice, actually many times, in the same place. As the storm continues, it may be very dangerous to approach the scene, especially if it is on a hilltop or cliff face. Look for more than one patient; a significant percentage of lightning incidents involve two or more people.

Risk Management

- Sit on an insulator to reduce contact with ground current
- Spread your group out to avoid a multiple casualty strike
- Inside a vehicle is best, on or under a vehicle is bad.
- If moving toward safety; keep moving
- Don't lean on a wire fence
- Lower is safer

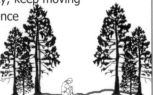

Treatment of Lightning Injury: While lightning is mythical, unpredictable, and poorly understood, the emergency treatment of lightning injury is not. Treat what you see. Remember that this is one of the rare cases in the field where a person in cardiopulmonary arrest might be saved by the quick application of CPR.

The burns caused by lightning tend to be superficial, but fluid loss can cause shock and hypothermia. In any large area burn, IV fluids and protection from heat loss are important. Shock, anticipated shock, head injury and ICP, and musculo-skeletal trauma are all treated as you would with any other patient.

Even if stabilized in the field, most lightning-strike patients should be evacuated for medical follow-up. Lightning-related problems can develop hours or days later. Evacuation need not be an emergency if there are no existing or anticipated critical system problems. ✚

Lightning Injuries

Scene Size-up:

- Scene is unsafe if storm continues.
- Multiple victims are likely.

Assessment and Treatment:

- Immediate Basic Life Support
- Treat what you see
- Evacuate for medical follow-up

"…the types of internal injures typical of household current are rarely seen with lightning."

Chapter 17

Avalanche Rescue

Predicting and avoiding avalanches is a topic worthy of its own text. As more people enter the backcountry for recreation, avalanche deaths in the United States are increasing sharply, particularly among snow machine operators. It is interesting to note that the vast majority of avalanche victims have some degree of avalanche awareness training.

In an avalanche burial the most important factor in survival is speed of recovery. In the first 15 minutes, 92 percent of victims are found alive. This drops to about 30 percent at 35 minutes, and around 3 percent at 130 minutes. It makes sense that most of the victims who survive are dug out by the people traveling with them, not by rescue teams arriving hours later.

In spite of this dim outlook, no one buried in an avalanche should be given up for dead based only on time. A few people have survived very long burials when trapped with an air pocket around a tree or in a vehicle or wrecked building. The record in the United States is twenty-two hours, and there are stories from Europe of people being found alive after days under the snow.

Avalanche Survival

Related to speed of recovery:

- 92% at 15 minutes of burial
- 30% at 35 minutes of burial
- 3% at 130 minutes of burial

Brugger and Falk

"It makes sense that most of the victims that survive are dug out by the people traveling with them, not by rescue teams arriving hours later."

The most efficient tool for locating a buried victim is a well-trained avalanche search dog team, but these rarely arrive on-scene soon enough to make a difference. If the victim is wearing an avalanche beacon, other members of the group may be able to perform a location and recover within minutes. Even then, the use of a beacon only increases your chance of survival by about 10 percent. If neither dog nor beacon is available, a live find is unlikely unless some part of the victim is projecting above the surface of the snow. The backup plan consists of a probe line of rescuers working slowly through the debris field.

There are a number of other devices being tested and used in avalanche recovery. Metal detectors are useful for locating snow machines or skis, which may or may not be near the buried victim. The Recco System used in some ski areas is a device that broadcasts a directional radio wave that excites a small metallic tag or sticker sewn into the skier's clothing. The "reflected" signal is picked up by the unit's receiver and can be followed directly back to the victim. The device has also been known to detect a reflected signal off cell phones, radios, and other metallic objects.

If a live victim is recovered, the primary medical problem will be respiratory arrest due to asphyxiation. This can occur as a result of snow packed into the nose and mouth, the formation of an ice mask, or restricted respiratory excursion due to the pressure of the snowpack.

Live Find

Treat what you see:

- Respiratory failure or arrest is likely to be the primary problem

- Hypothermia is unlikely unless survivor has been buried for hours

- Once recovered, hypothermia is an anticipated problem

- Increased ICP is an anticipated problem from trauma and/or hypoxia

---

Snow is mostly air and is very porous. Unless the airway is packed with snow, the victim may be able to breathe for a period of time. Eventually, the victim's exhaled breath will condense and freeze into a nonporous ice mask around the airway. This effect may be delayed by the use of an Avalung™ or the good fortune to have large air space formed by vegetation or debris. For these reasons, an avalanche recovery is still considered an urgent response even if it will take a rescue team an hour or more to reach the scene.

The treatment includes immediate PPV, supplemental oxygen, and evacuation. Once the patient is freed from the snowpack, hypothermia becomes an anticipated problem. Airway control is critical if the patient is less than A on AVPU. Increased intracranial pressure due to brain hypoxia can also develop, but this is likely to occur well after an evacuation has been accomplished.

The resuscitation of an avalanche victim in full cardiopulmonary arrest should not be attempted if there are obvious lethal injuries or the effort puts rescuers at risk. Experience shows that the chances of success are minimal after thirty minutes of complete burial. If the victim's airway is packed with snow, you can assume that breathing stopped at the time the avalanche occurred. If you choose to begin CPR the effort may be discontinued after thirty minutes of sustained cardiac arrest. ✚

Chapter 18

Arthropod Disease Vectors

Ticks

Ticks themselves are not much of a problem. They mind their own business, cause no pain, eat very little, and depart quietly when they're done. Not bad for a biting arthropod.

But like lots of other creatures, ticks carry disease. Current favorites include Rocky Mountain spotted fever, Colorado tick fever, tick paralysis, and Lyme disease. These present with a constellation of confusing symptoms and are not easy to diagnose.

It is much easier to avoid contracting the disease in the first place, and this means avoiding ticks. Experts on the subject recommend wearing a long-sleeved shirt with long pants tucked into high socks, and a bandanna high on the neck under a low hat. Apply insect repellent to clothing, especially around cuff and neck openings, and on exposed skin. By following these recommendations, you will reduce the chance of feeding a tick and acquiring a tick-borne disease. You will also be sweating bullets, smell like a toxic waste dump, and look twice as scary as the fashion models in the sporting goods catalogs.

Another option is to get into the habit of frequently looking for them on your skin and clothing. They usually like to crawl around for a while before settling in to feed. Frequent inspections will get rid of most of them before they attach themselves. Already attached ticks can be removed by gently prying them off with tweezers. Sometimes the mouthparts will break off and be left in the skin. Try to scrape these out with a sharp blade or needle. Prompt removal of ticks will help prevent the spread of disease. Lyme disease, for example, is not effectively transmitted until the tick has been in place for a day or so. Unfortunately, Rocky Mountain spotted fever can be transmitted in just a few hours.

You should not attempt removal by burning the tick or suffocating or poisoning it with petroleum jelly, alcohol, gasoline, or mineral oil. This may cause the tick to regurgitate infectious material into the bite. Do not handle the tick without gloves or other protection.

"Tick country" is vegetated: woods, grass, and brush. Tick season is spring, summer, and fall. Adult ticks are eight-legged arthropods ranging in size from nearly microscopic to a centimeter in diameter. The ticks of greatest concern are 2 to 4 mm in diameter and, before they begin to feed, are easily recognized as a foreign creature on your skin. Once attached and engorged with blood, they look more like a wart, mole, or other skin part, and may be missed by someone who doesn't know your body as well as you do.

The appearance of flulike symptoms, rash, and muscular aches and pains several days to weeks after a confirmed tick attachment is well worth bringing to the attention of a medical practitioner. These illnesses can be quite a diagnostic dilemma with a variety of neurological symptoms, fevers, and aches and pains. If you saved the tick, bring it with you. Some ticks can be tested for diseases like Lyme.

Tick-borne Disease

Prevention:

- DEET or Picardin on skin
- Permethrin on clothing
- Tight weave clothing
- Frequent tick checks
- Prompt removal of attached ticks
- Post Exposure Prophylaxis in Lyme endemic regions

"Tick country is vegetated: woods, grass, and brush. Tick season is spring, summer, and fall."

Mosquitoes

The list of diseases transmitted by mosquitoes includes malaria, filariasis, West Nile virus, equine encephalitis, and a host of others. The key to avoiding these infections is to avoid being a host to mosquitoes. Like ticks, they can be deterred by insect repellent and tight-weave clothing. Unlike ticks, they can transmit disease in less than a minute.

Prophylactic medication can help prevent or treat malaria infection. However, some diseases like filariasis have no effective cure or drugs to prevent them. Preventing exposure is your only defense.

The best insect repellents for ticks and mosquitoes currently available include DEET, permethrin, and picardin. DEET and permethrin are both extensively studied and are considered safe and effective. DEET can be used on the exposed skin of hands, ankles, and the face. There is no advantage to using a formulation greater than 35 percent DEET. Permethrin is recommended for clothing and has been shown to remain effective after twenty or more washings.

Fleas and Lice

Only about 5 percent of a given flea population is actively feeding on blood. The rest are in various stages of development as eggs, pupae, and larvae. Adult fleas can hibernate for up to two years waiting for a blood meal.

The worst place to sleep is on that old mattress in the trekking hut that was last occupied six weeks ago. The eggs, pupae, and larvae have matured and are waiting for you. Only a few of them need to be carrying the bacterium *Yersinia pestis* to give you bubonic plague. Fleas can be killed or deterred by insect repellents and insecticides. Your own sleeping bag, frequently washed, is another good defense.

Lice are easily transmitted between people sharing clothing and furniture. The adults are easily killed with permethrin or malathione. Reapplication may be necessary in ten days to kill the newly hatched larvae. In the absence of permethrin shampoo, lice can also be smothered with a layer of any viscous substance like petroleum jelly or mayonnaise. It may not be pretty, but it can solve your problem! ✚

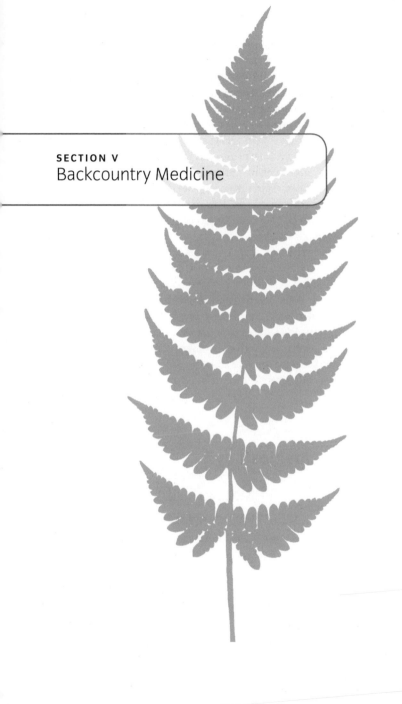

Chapter 19
A General Approach to Illness

As a medical practitioner, I much prefer trauma to illness. Something which is merely broken or torn usually presents a straightforward mechanical problem. Illness is often confusing and scary and defies a quick fix. The nonspecific symptoms of many illnesses generate a long list of possible diagnoses. In the emergency department setting, it can be very difficult to figure out exactly what you're dealing with. In the backcountry it can be impossible. Our working diagnosis may remain as generic as "serious" or "not serious."

An Approach to Illness

- Critical system problem?
- Ins and outs?
- Pain?
- Mental status?
- Serious or not serious?

"Even in the emergency department, it can be difficult to figure out exactly what you're dealing with. Our working diagnosis may remain as generic as *serious*, or *not serious*.

There is little value in leafing through lists of symptoms and descriptions of diseases just so you can put a name on your patient's problem. The laboratory and X-ray aren't available to confirm your suspicions anyway. Your primary job in dealing with illness is to keep your patient safe, comfortable, and well hydrated, and to watch for the development of anything serious. The human body is a remarkable organism and will heal itself just fine in the vast majority of cases.

As you evaluate an illness, beware of focusing too much attention on the numbers. By all means, take vital signs, but don't forget to look at the patient. Their behavior is more important than their statistics. We worry much more about a confused and lethargic person with a temperature of 37.5 degrees C, than an active and oriented patient with a fever of 40 degrees C.

A healthy person willingly takes in food and fluid and produces urine and feces in more or less proportional amounts. She is interested in her surroundings and knows who she is and what she's doing there. She will freely move, dress, and protect herself from the environment.

A patient who is ill but basically okay may be grumpy and uncomfortable but will continue to eat and drink and function more or less normally. You don't need to worry about him too much. It is when your patient stops eating and drinking, loses interest in his surroundings, and is unable to take care of himself that you should consider the situation serious. This is the time to be looking for expert help, regardless of the diagnosis. ✚

Chapter 20

Abdominal Pain

The word abdomen is a derivation of Latin for "hidden," and rightly so. Everything that goes on inside the abdomen is well hidden from our eyes and can become the subject of a lot of conjecture and consternation. How do you know if your crew member's belly pain is from a developing appendicitis, or an underdeveloped ability to digest whole grains? Should you call a passing ship for a lift back to Portland, or stick it out until you reach Bermuda?

Few symptoms can cause as much unnecessary grief as abdominal pain. Even experienced surgeons using a variety of diagnostic tests and tools have a difficult time figuring out what's going on inside a sore abdomen. Don't feel too bad if you can't figure it out either. Focus instead on the *one* important question: Is this abdominal pain serious or not serious?

Abdominal Pain

- *Gastroenteritis*
- *Ectopic pregnancy*
- *Appendicitis*
- *Cholecystitis*
- *Diverticulitis*
- *Perforating ulcer*
- *Pancreatitis*
- *Etc.*

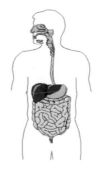

Serious or Not Serious?

For our purposes, we can consider the abdomen to be hiding three major components: hollow organs, solid organs, and the sensitive abdominal lining called the peritoneum. Hollow structures, like the stomach, intestines, and gall bladder, contain digestive fluids and have muscular walls that contract rhythmically to move these fluids along the digestive system. The ureters and urinary bladder use similar structure and function to contain and move urine from the kidneys to the outside.

Solid organs have a variety of functions and associated diseases, but we worry mostly about their potential for rupture in abdominal trauma. The liver, spleen, and kidneys are part of the body core and are richly supplied with blood. These structures can split open like a watermelon dropped from a truck, and bleeding can be severe.

The peritoneum is a membrane that lines all of the organs and the abdominal wall inside the body cavity. It is exquisitely sensitive to irritation from things like blood, bacteria, and digestive fluids that have gotten loose inside the cavity as a result of injury or illness. The peritoneum also represents a large surface area (greater than your skin) which, when inflamed, can leak a large volume of fluid in a short period of time.

The nerve cells in hollow organs transmit pain sensations primarily when stretched, like when you distend your stomach with a big Thanksgiving dinner. The pain of distention gets worse when the organ system attempts its normal, rhythmic muscular contractions.

The kind of abdominal pain we usually don't worry about is caused by the intermittent stretching of the hollow organs of the digestive system. The mechanism is usually gas, fluid, and spasm created by a viral illness, food intolerance, or constipation. The pain is the generalized, crampy type that precedes a bout of diarrhea or flatulence, after which you feel a whole lot better. The problem is well contained within the intestine and, when relieved, the system returns to normal. This kind of abdominal pain is usually associated with conditions that might be unpleasant but are not serious.

Real problems begin when whatever is happening inside the gut begins to irritate the peritoneal lining inside of the abdomen. Unlike hollow organ pain, peritoneal pain is location-specific and constant rather than crampy. Movement makes it worse as the inflamed membranes rub against each other.

In the classic case of appendicitis, for example, the problem begins with the obstruction of the appendix, which is a part of the hollow intestine in the lower right quadrant of the abdomen. As you know, obstruction ultimately leads to infection and swelling. The early symptoms are often the generalized, crampy discomfort typical of hollow organ stretching, and you would probably not label it as serious.

As the infection develops, the swollen and inflamed appendix will begin to irritate the peritoneal lining of the intestine and abdomen. The symptoms will begin to change from generalized cramping to localized constant pain in the right lower quadrant. If the condition gets bad enough, the organ will burst, spilling digestive enzymes and pus into the abdominal cavity. At that point, the whole peritoneum becomes inflamed, with swelling and fluid leakage. Shock and death are almost inevitable.

The key to early recognition of this serious problem is the change in character of the pain from crampy and generalized to constant and localized. The same is true of other hollow organ problems like cholecystitis (gall bladder infection), ectopic pregnancy (fetus in the fallopian tube), and bowel obstruction. It is not necessary to know exactly what you're dealing with to know that it needs a surgeon and an operating room.

Solid organs like the liver have few nerve endings that sense pain. Most of the discomfort with solid organ problems comes from irritation of the organ's peritoneal lining due to infection or bleeding. Both are serious. Blunt trauma with a ruptured solid organ can lead to shock, which should be anticipated in cases of persistent abdominal pain following injury. Again, pain tends to be localized and constant.

Another common source of abdominal discomfort following trauma or exertion is pain in the muscles of the abdominal wall. This is not associated with any internal organs and is not serious but can be difficult to distinguish from peritoneal irritation. This type of pain will usually be relieved by rest and made worse by use of the injured muscles.

If vomiting or diarrhea is a component of the problem, you need to be thinking about volume shock from dehydration. This is a big killer of young children and older patients, especially with diseases like cholera. In the backcountry rehydration can be difficult or impossible.

Diagramming and discussing all of the possible causes of abdominal pain would quadruple the size of this book but still not help you much in the backcountry or far out to sea. Even if you could tell an ectopic pregnancy from appendicitis, you're not going to haul out your fillet knife and operate on either one. What you really want to know is serious or not serious, evacuate or wait and watch? The following "red flag" symptoms should help in your decision.

Abdominal Pain

Red Flags:

- Constant, localized pain and tenderness
- Aggravated by movement and palpation
- Persistent fever
- Bloody vomit or diarrhea
- Tachycardia
- Lasts more than 24 hours

Treatment of Abdominal Pain: Treat the cause. This usually means that you can't fix it in the field. Whether you're a surgeon or a woodcutter, red flags mean evacuation. You should continue to monitor the patient during transport and note any changes in condition. In the long-term-care setting, abdominal pain or the accompanying red flags may resolve, revealing the problem to be less serious. It's always better to cancel or slow down an evacuation in progress rather than to start one too late.

Give fluids to make up for normal and abnormal losses. This is best restricted to water and rehydration solutions. We know that surgeons and anesthesiologists would prefer a patient with an empty stomach, but maintaining fluid volume is critical to survival in the long-term-care situation.

Oral pain medication should be restricted to acetaminophen because other anti-inflammatory drugs can irritate the gut. Injectable pain medication is preferable. See also the related topics of vomiting, diarrhea, constipation, and dehydration. ✚

Serious Abdominal Pain

Anticipate:

- Volume shock
- Systemic infection

Treatment:

- Maintain hydration
- Maintain body core temperature
- Restrict foods to easily absorbed sugars
- Emergency evacuation

Chapter 21

Chest Pain

Just about anybody who enters a hospital emergency department and uses the words "chest" and "pain" in the same sentence gets evaluated for heart attack. This is almost instinctive, even though medical practitioners know that there are many causes of chest pain that have nothing to do with the heart. They recognize that the risk and expense involved in testing for heart attack is much lower than the risk and expense involved in failing to detect one. For the hospital, the choice is easy and the policy is clear. Unfortunately, this does not translate very well to the remote environment. We need a much better indication that the pain is the result of a serious problem to balance against the hazards of evacuation.

Chest Pain

- *Myocardial ischemia*
- *Stable angina*
- *Respiratory infection*
- *Chest wall muscle strain*
- *Chest wall contusion*
- *Esophageal spasm*
- *Pulmonary embolus*
- *Etc.*

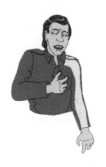

Serious or Not Serious?

Just like the hospital, we look for a reasonable explanation for the pain, and this may include ischemic heart muscle. Often, however, it can be attributed to one of a number of other possibilities. The most common in the backcountry setting is muscle or rib pain from exercise or injury. This type of pain can usually be reproduced by movement. There is often a tender area in the same spot that the patient complains of pain. It is usually relieved by rest and aspirin or ibuprofen. The patient does not usually appear otherwise sick or short of breath.

Chest pain from respiratory infection or lung injury will usually have a pretty clear history of preceding illness. It may be accompanied by cough, fever, and sore throat. It is usually made worse by coughing and deep breathing. The patient is usually somewhat ill in appearance. This pain may be part of a serious respiratory system problem, but not an indication of heart attack.

The pain associated with indigestion is usually accompanied by burping, heartburn, and nausea. Unlike the pain of heart attack, it is often relieved by antacids. The patient will often give a long-standing history of similar episodes associated with certain foods or stress.

The chest pain of a heart attack is caused by ischemia (inadequate perfusion) of the heart muscle due to spasm or clotting of the coronary (heart) arteries. It is typically described as being in the middle of the chest radiating to the jaw and left arm. The pain is often referred to as "crushing or constricting." There may be shortness of breath and sweating. In a few cases, vital signs will show an irregular heartbeat and the signs of shock (cardiogenic shock). At least this is what the textbook says.

Unfortunately, the classic pattern does not occur in all cases of heart attack. It can be mistaken for indigestion, respiratory infection, or chest wall pain. In fact, the patient will be trying very hard to mistake it for anything but heart attack. If there is no other obvious cause, we must consider the possibility that the chest pain is due to myocardial ischemia. This is more likely when the patient has some of the risk factors associated with heart disease.

Serious Chest Pain
Heart Attack

Risk Factors:

- Hypertension
- High blood cholesterol
- Male over 40 years old
- Post menopausal female
- Smoking, obesity, diabetes
- Family or personal history of heart disease
- Recreational use of amphetamines or cocaine

This does not mean that your slim, nonsmoking, athletic, twenty-year-old girlfriend can't have heart problems. It just means that it is very unlikely, and you are not going to call for a heroic evacuation with that thought in mind.

But if your chest pain patient is your overweight, two-pack-a-day smoking, fifty-five-year-old law firm partner, you'd best get him out of the woods. This does not mean he *is* having a heart attack, but the likelihood is high enough to justify evacuation.

Treatment of Suspected Heart Attack: "Time is myocardium" is the mantra of treatment. The sooner the ischemia can be reversed, the less heart muscle will be damaged and the better the chance for survival. This means an urgent evacuation begun the moment that you decide that you are dealing with serious chest pain.

The ideal evacuation would not increase the stress or level of exertion for your patient. But you may find yourself choosing between a walk-out evacuation that takes an hour and a carry-out that may take several hours. You should favor the route that will put your patient under advanced life support care as soon as possible while causing the least increase in activity and oxygen demand.

As long as your patient is not already taking blood-thinning medications, give one adult aspirin tablet by mouth. This will reduce the tendency of the blood to clot, which may reduce ischemia in the heart muscle. If the patient has other heart medication, like nitroglycerine, assist him in taking it according to directions. Advise any rescue teams responding to your situation to bring oxygen. ✚

Heart Attack

Field Treatment:

- Assist with nitroglycerin as prescribed
- Give one adult aspirin
- PROP
- Gentle but expeditious evacuation:
  - activity increases myocardial oxygen demand
  - time increases infarction
- ALS care as soon as possible

Chapter 22

Diarrhea

One of the functions of the large intestine is to absorb fluid from feces just before excretion. This serves to conserve the body's fluid balance and allow you some degree of control over when and where excretion occurs. Diarrhea develops when the lining of the intestinal space is irritated by infection or toxins and fails to absorb fluid. The intestine can, in addition, leak more body fluid on its own, contributing to general fluid loss.

Like abdominal pain, what we want to know is serious or not serious? Diarrhea that is a softer version of normal stool and relatively infrequent is usually nothing to worry about. Even if it lasts for several days or weeks, fluid losses can be replaced by oral intake.

Diarrhea can be a symptom of other more serious problems, especially in the presence of abdominal pain. Diarrhea itself becomes a real problem when fluid loss occurs so rapidly that it cannot be replaced by drinking and eating.

Diarrhea

Red Flags:

- Associated with red flags for abdominal pain
- Fluid losses exceed intake
- Persistent fever
- Bloody diarrhea
- Signs of shock

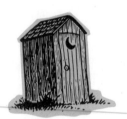

Treatment of Diarrhea: Diarrhea that does not show red flag signs can sometimes be helped by bismuth subsalicylate (brand: Pepto Bismol) or similar over-the-counter preparations. Beware of drugs such as loperamide (brand: Imodium) that inhibit intestinal motility, especially in the presence of fever. If the cause of the diarrhea is an intestinal bacteria or parasite, obstructing drainage can increase the severity of the infection.

Most importantly, you should pay attention to replacing fluid losses with oral electrolyte solutions or just water and bland food. Time will usually correct the situation, but if the problem persists longer than a week, medical advice should be sought.

When red flag signs are noted, evacuation should be considered. If signs of volume shock are present, evacuation should be urgent if fluids cannot be replaced quickly in the field. During evacuation, oral fluids should be given as quickly as the patient can tolerate. ✚

Diarrhea

Anticipate:

- Volume shock from dehydration

Treatment:

- Fluid and easily absorbed food
- Preserve body core temperature
- Loperamide (Imodium) if no red flags (4 mg x 1 dose, then 2 mg after each loose stool)
- Bismuth subsalicylate (Pepto-Bismol)
- Antibiotics for traveler's diarrhea

Chapter 23
Constipation

Constipation is usually the result of the large intestine doing just what it's supposed to do, absorb fluid from feces. If you are dehydrated, fluid recovery can turn feces into something resembling metamorphic rock. This can be tough for even the most energetic hollow organ muscle contractions to deal with. This is definitely a problem worth an effort at prevention.

Maintaining fluid balance by staying well hydrated will make it unnecessary for the large intestine to absorb too much fluid from feces. A good indicator for hydration is urine production. You should be drinking enough fluid to be producing light-yellow–colored urine frequently.

Take the time and find the privacy for a decent bowel movement. This is especially difficult on boats at sea in rough conditions or on a big wall climb when relieving oneself becomes a life-threatening adventure. Nevertheless, it is extremely important. If feces sit in the intestine long enough, metamorphosis will occur no matter how well hydrated you are.

Diets high in fiber create bulk, which stimulates bowel contraction and retains water in the fecal material. If you are condemned by circumstance to a high-protein diet or dehydrated food, consider taking fiber capsules along on the trip (brand: Metamucil Gel Caps). Two per day can simulate the effect of a salad with every meal. Taking the pills with salad dressing can almost make it seem real.

Constipation becomes annoying when you feel bad because of it. Constipation becomes a problem when the rest of the body begins to suffer. Exactly when this occurs is highly individual. We have had students go nine days before mentioning the lack of a bowel movement, while others become cranky after only twenty-four hours.

Treatment of Constipation: Hydration is the best initial treatment and will often solve the problem. The next step is the use of a stool softener like senna (brand: Senokot) or docusate sodium (brand: Colace). Mineral oil taken orally as an intestinal lubricant can reduce friction and allow stool to move. These treatments are very mild and generally very safe.

Laxatives like bisacodyl (brand: Dulcolax) given orally or by suppository stimulate the bowel to contract. This is most effective and least painful after hydration and the administration of a stool softener. Laxatives can be dangerous if the patient has a bowel obstruction. Do not use these drugs in the presence of red flags for abdominal pain.

An enema is viewed by most people as the treatment of last resort. Warm water is instilled into the rectum by gravity feed. A small amount may be all that is necessary to lubricate and soften stool. An enema is also contraindicated with the red flags for abdominal pain. ✚

Constipation

Anticipate:

- Serious abdominal pain
- Systemic infection

Treatment:

- Hydration
- Stool softeners; Colace, Senokot
- Laxatives*; Dulcolax, Ex-lax
- Enema*

* Not in the presence of serious abdominal pain.

Chapter 24

Nausea and Vomiting

Like diarrhea, vomiting can be the result of a problem with the gastrointestinal system, or be a symptom of other problems such as motion sickness, toxic ingestion, increasing intracranial pressure, or infection. Finding and treating the primary cause is the priority. However, you must consider the additional problems that can be caused by severe fluid loss as well.

Vomiting associated with red flags is considered serious. This includes sea sickness that is persistent and not responsive to medication, or persistent vomiting for any reason.

Vomiting

Red Flags:

- Cannot control airway
- Cannot replace fluids
- Cannot maintain calories and body core temp
- Associated with red flags for abdominal pain

"Airway obstruction and aspiration is an anticipated problem in any vomiting patient. Position and constant monitoring is critical if the patient is not A and oriented…"

Treatment of Vomiting: Maintaining hydration is a priority. Because giving fluids by mouth will be difficult, intravenous or rectal rehydration may be necessary. Oral intake may be successful if the patient can take small amounts frequently enough to maintain hydration. Look for normal urine output as evidence of success.

Airway obstruction and aspiration is an anticipated problem in any vomiting patient. Position and constant monitoring is critical if the patient is not A and oriented on the AVPU scale. Aspiration of vomit into the lungs carries about a 20 percent mortality rate.

Antiemetic drugs can be given by intramuscular or intravenous injection, or by rectal suppository. The prescription drugs promethazine, compazine, and trimethobenzamide are examples. The over-the-counter antihistamines meclizine and diphenhydramine can be effective if the patient can tolerate oral medication. Acetaminophen is preferred over NSAIDs or oral narcotics for pain.

There are many antiemetic drugs. One of the most common and useful is Benadryl (diphenhydramine), which is also used for allergy and cold symptoms. Being able to give drugs by rectal suppository is a real advantage in persistent vomiting. Phenergan or Tigan suppositories might be a good addition to an expedition medical kit. Please consult a medical practitioner. ✚

Vomiting

Anticipate:

- Airway obstruction and aspiration
- Volume shock from dehydration

Treatment:

- Airway control
- Hydration and calories
- Maintain body core temperature
- Anti-emetic medication

Chapter 25
Ear and Sinus Problems

Swimmer's Ear (External Otitis)

Swimmer's ear is an inflammation of the external auditory canal, that is, the tube leading from the outside environment to the outside surface of the eardrum. The problem is usually caused by bacteria that invade skin softened by prolonged soaking in water.

Like any infection, it will be characterized by redness, warmth, swelling, and pain. The external structures of the ear and surrounding area will be tender to touch, and the ear canal itself will be exquisitely sensitive. There is usually a history of recent and repetitive immersion in water.

Treatment of Swimmer's Ear: The treatment of choice is antibiotic ear drops, available by physician's prescription. In lieu of that, regular cleansing of the ear canal with rubbing alcohol followed by mineral oil should reduce the amount of debris and bacteria and contribute to healing. Do not use dry cotton swabs because they will further irritate the ear canal. Staying out of the water and allowing the ear to heal will help considerably.

Middle Ear Infection and Sinusitis

The area referred to as the "middle ear" begins inside the eardrum and extends through a narrow opening into the nasal cavity. It is similar in structure to the other sinuses, which are open spaces, lined by mucous membranes, with narrow openings into the nose. Middle ear infection and sinusitis are good examples of the obstruction to infection principle. The usual cause is swelling and inflammation from a viral infection, or exposure to water when swimming. The obstructed space fills with fluid, which becomes colonized by bacteria.

The typical sign of sinus infection is facial or ear pain. There will often be a history of several days of mild cold or flu symptoms with a stuffy or runny nose. Bending over at the waist increases pressure in the affected sinus or ear and increases the pain. Sinusitis, in the form of middle ear infection, can be differentiated from swimmer's ear by the fact that, although the ear hurts, the external ear structures and ear canal are not red, swollen, or tender to touch. In more severe infections you may see some discharge of green or yellow pus from the nose or from the ear if the eardrum ruptures. Fever is another symptom of more serious infection.

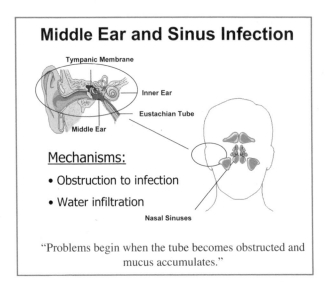

Middle Ear and Sinus Infection

Tympanic Membrane

Inner Ear

Eustachian Tube

Middle Ear

Nasal Sinuses

Mechanisms:

- Obstruction to infection
- Water infiltration

"Problems begin when the tube becomes obstructed and mucus accumulates."

Red flags for middle ear and sinus infection reflect the anticipated problems of inner ear involvement or systemic infection. Persistent fever, severe pain, or altered mental status all may indicate a serious condition and warrant emergency evacuation. Vertigo, the sense of spinning and disequilibrium, may indicate inner ear involvement. This should also be considered serious.

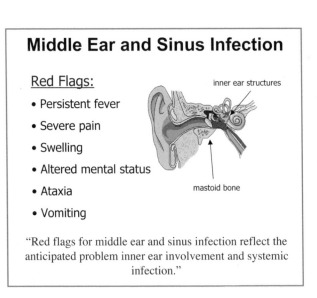

Middle Ear and Sinus Infection

Red Flags:

- Persistent fever
- Severe pain
- Swelling
- Altered mental status
- Ataxia
- Vomiting

inner ear structures

mastoid bone

"Red flags for middle ear and sinus infection reflect the anticipated problem inner ear involvement and systemic infection."

Treatment of Middle Ear Infection and Sinusitis: Like any obstructed space, it can be improved by drainage. A middle ear infection may drain spontaneously through a weak point in the eardrum, which is actually a natural protective mechanism. If pain is relieved and no fever develops, there is no emergency in this. Keep the ear dry and see your doctor when you get ashore.

We can try to reduce the swelling that is causing the obstruction of the narrow sinus openings by using decongestant nasal spray, or having the patient breathe steam from a pot of hot water. Systemic decongestants such as pseudoephedrine (brand: Sudafed) tablets will also help. Keeping your patient well hydrated is important. This will keep mucus from drying and becoming too thick to drain. Antibiotics are often necessary for complete treatment if the infection is well established. ✚

Middle Ear and Sinus Infection

Anticipate:

- Pain
- Spread of infection

Treatment:

- OTC decongestants
- Inhaled steam
- Saline irrigation
- Antibiotics if symptoms persist

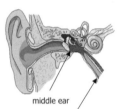

middle ear

Eustachian tube

"… the situation can be improved with drainage."

It doesn't take much trauma to rupture the blood vessels in the nose. The most easily injured ones are near the front of the nose. Bleeding from here will drain out of the nose if the patient is positioned upright with the head forward.

The task here is to distinguish a simple nosebleed from something more serious. If the bleeding started spontaneously, or while blowing or picking your nose, you can be pretty sure it's not complicated. However, if the bleed is the result of trauma, you must consider the possibility of facial bone fracture.

Nosebleed

Treatment:

- Direct pressure (squeeze nostrils x 15 minutes)
- Nasal tampon with vasoconstrictor (Afrin)
- Clot-enhancing powders

Red Flags:

- Associated fever, infection, or TBI
- Profuse and persistent bleeding

Treatment of Nosebleed: First, calm your patient and have her sit down. Position her to allow for drainage out of the nose, and have her blow out any clots. This sounds scary, but it won't cause the bleeding to get worse. Now, you or the patient should pinch the nostrils together and hold firmly *for fifteen minutes* while sitting upright. This applies simple direct pressure to the most likely bleeding source. Remember, to stop the bleeding it is essential to hold enough pressure for a long enough time. This should stop most of the nosebleeds that you are likely to see.

A persistent anterior bleed can be treated for a longer period by inserting a small tampon into the nostril and wetting it with a decongestant like Afrin or Dristan. These are topical vasoconstrictors that will reduce bleeding just as they keep your nose from producing too much mucus. The patient will look pretty funny with a string hanging out of his nose, but the tampon can be left in place safely for a couple of hours.

Clot-enhancing powders have also found a place in treating nosebleeds. These substances are generally ineffective for the life-threatening bleeding for which they were originally marketed, but do fine with minor nuisance bleeding. Typically, a small amount of powder is supplied with a cotton swab for application.

A large amount of blood running down the throat from the back of the nose is also a sign of a potentially serious posterior bleed. This is of special concern if the patient is taking blood-thinning medication, even aspirin. These can be difficult to control without posterior nasal packing. The patient is at risk for shock, vomiting, and airway obstruction.

Your best response is the same as for any other bleeding that you are unable to control. Make the patient comfortable and prepare for an evacuation. If the patient needs to lie down, protect the airway by positioning her facedown or on her side with the chest and head supported to allow for drainage from the nose and mouth. A carry-out evacuation may be necessary. ✚

Chapter 27
Urinary Tract Infection

The female urethra is only a few centimeters long. It is fairly easy for normal skin surface or intestinal bacteria to migrate from the outside into the normally sterile bladder. Once there, bacteria are able to reproduce rapidly and begin to invade and inflame the soft tissue lining. Normally, frequent urination flushes bacteria out of the bladder and urethra, preventing this from happening.

In both the civilized and backcountry settings, there are a number of ways that this system can be upset. Perhaps the most common to the wilderness traveler is urinary retention. This is usually due to slight dehydration. The body's normal efforts to preserve fluid results in low urine output and infrequent flushing of the urinary tract. The same situation can occur simply through lack of opportunity to urinate, such as "holding it" until morning rather than getting out of a warm sleeping bag in the middle of the night. Either way, any bacteria entering the bladder and urethra have a longer period of time in which to multiply and invade the tissue lining.

Another common cause of urinary tract infection in the female is inadequate hygiene. In settings where bathing is difficult or impossible, the number of bacteria on the outer surface of the skin increases dramatically. Add this to the habit of "drip drying" instead of using toilet paper and you have a greater opportunity for infection.

A third mechanism for infection is direct trauma to the urethra. The usual culprit is frequent or vigorous sexual activity, but it can also be caused by the saddle of a mountain bike or a climbing harness. This is the so-called honeymoon cystitis. The urethral opening becomes inflamed, is invaded by bacteria, and infection results.

More complicated and dangerous infections can develop when the bacteria climb beyond the bladder to invade the ureters and kidney. Sexually transmitted diseases are also considered more dangerous because the bacteria or virus is foreign to the body and is more difficult to eradicate. In the male, because the urethra is so much longer, infection of the urinary tract is unusual and always indicates a complicated condition. The most common cause is sexually transmitted disease.

The classic symptoms of uncomplicated urinary tract infection include low pelvic pain, frequent urination in small amounts, cloudy or blood-tinged urine, and pain, tingling, or burning on urination. In the female it is possible to confuse infection of the urinary tract with vaginal infection. Inflammation of the vagina and external genitalia can also cause pain and burning on urination (see vaginitis).

Symptoms that indicate infection has progressed beyond the superficial lining of the urethra and bladder can include any of the symptoms above plus the following red flags:

Urinary Tract Infection

Red Flags:

- Male
- Back pain (kidney involvement)
- Fever (systemic infection)
- Serious abdominal pain
- Bloody urine
- Known sexually transmitted disease

"Antibiotic therapy and urgent evacuation are indicated."

Treatment of Urinary Tract Infection: The treatment for uncomplicated urinary tract infection usually includes the use of antibiotics and hydration. Temporary measures, pending access to medical care, involve treating UTI like any other soft tissue infection with drainage and cleansing. Keep the external genitalia as clean as possible. Drink plenty of fluids to irrigate the infection.

Symptoms of UTI accompanied by red flags indicate a potentially serious problem. These include fever, back pain, and blood in the urine. The possibility of sexually transmitted disease should also be considered a red flag. Antibiotic therapy and urgent evacuation are indicated. Infection of the kidneys is a life-threatening condition. ✚

Urinary Tract Infection

Mechanisms:

- Obstruction
- Dehydration
- Inadequate hygiene
- Localized trauma.

Treatment:

- Hydration
- Antibiotics

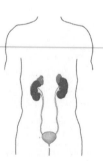

Chapter 28
Vaginitis

Inflammation and infection of the vagina often occur when something upsets the normal ecological balance between yeast and bacteria, allowing one of the species to grow out of control. For example, taking penicillin for a strep throat will kill many of the bacteria in the vagina as well. This opens the way for an overgrowth of yeast, which is not affected by penicillin. Changes in the vaginal environment caused by clothing, sexual activity, stress, and other factors can upset this balance as well.

Yeast infection is more common than bacterial vaginitis. Signs and symptoms of yeast infection include itching or burning and a whitish or "cheesy" vaginal discharge. There may also be tingling or burning as urine irritates inflamed tissues, causing some confusion with urinary tract infection.

Bacterial vaginitis also causes itching and burning, but the discharge is typically yellow or brown and malodorous. A lost tampon is a common cause. Medication use, diabetes, and other systemic problems can also contribute.

Vaginitis becomes serious when it migrates into the uterus and fallopian tubes, causing the infection known as pelvic inflammatory disease. The symptoms will include the easily recognized red flags for abdominal pain. Sexually transmitted disease should also be considered serious.

Treatment of Vaginitis: Needless to say, suspected pelvic inflammatory disease warrants evacuation to medical care. Simple yeast vaginitis may respond to non-prescription treatment in the field. Bacterial vaginitis generally requires antibiotics.

Vaginitis

Mechanisms:

- Antibiotics
- Obstruction to infection (occlusive clothing)
- Sexual activity
- Inadequate hygiene
- Overgrowth of yeast or bacteria

"Infection of the vagina occurs when something upsets
the normal balance between yeast and bacteria..."

Vaginitis

Signs and Symptoms:

- Yeast - white, cheesy discharge
- Bacterial - yellow/brown, malodorous discharge
- Itchy, burning sensation on contact with urine

Red Flags:

- Associated with red flags for abdominal pain
- Pregnancy

"Many women presenting with yeast vaginitis will have a previous history of similar symptoms, and will recognize the problem and know the treatment."

Treatment:

- Yeast Infection:
    - fluconazole tablet (Diflucan, Rx)
    - topical antifungal (Monistat)
    - 1% PI douche x 3 days
- Bacterial Vaginitis:
    - oral or vaginal antibiotics
    - 1% PI douche x 3 days
    - evacuation for medical evaluation

If medical care is not available, a temporary reduction of symptoms, or a complete cure, can be achieved by using a douche made by diluting a teaspoon of povidone iodine solution in a quart of water once a day for several days. An alternative douche solution may be prepared by diluting a tablespoon of vinegar in a quart of water. A douche should not be used by a pregnant patient.

Nonprescription medications like clotrimazole cream or suppositories (brand: Lotrimin) are available for common yeast infections. The manufacturers warn against relying on this treatment unless the patient is fairly certain of the diagnosis through past experience. Because yeast and bacteria grow well in a warm and moist environment, the situation can also be improved by staying dry and cool. This means wearing loose-fitting clothing and spending less time in the wet suit. ✚

The "common cold" with its stuffy nose, sore throat, runny eyes, and cough has been harassing people since people began. There is no reason to believe that it won't pick on you, expedition or no expedition. You should be ready to deal with it.

The mild respiratory infections that we label "colds" or "flu" are caused by viruses. They produce a multiplicity of symptoms that conspire to keep us miserable until our body's immune system identifies the bug, produces specific antibodies, and eradicates it. Problems develop when the virus is particularly virulent, or the viral infection opens the way for a secondary bacterial infection to take hold. This is how people who start with a cold can end up with a bacterial pneumonia, bronchitis, or strep throat.

Respiratory Infection

Red Flags:

- Respiratory distress
- Significant difficulty swallowing secretions
- Persistent fever
- Bloody sputum
- Tachycardia
- Persistent chest pain

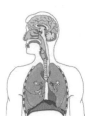

Mild upper respiratory infection is characterized by runny nose, mild headache, sneezing, coughing, irritated eyes, mild sore throat, muscular aches, and intermittent fever. Other than being slightly annoyed and uncomfortable, the patient is usually not significantly impaired in her ability to perform normal tasks, eat, and drink.

More serious respiratory disease may start with the above symptoms or develop independently. Coughing typically becomes productive of thick yellow, green, or brown sputum. The patient may experience chills, shortness of breath, and chest pain on respiration. Fever will be more persistent.

Any respiratory infection that is causing respiratory distress is no longer mild. Neither is an infection that interferes with eating and drinking. People with chronic respiratory problems like asthma are more likely to develop complications. These points should help you answer the all-important question: serious or not serious?

Treatment of Upper Respiratory Infection: The treatment of mild upper respiratory infection involves making the patient more comfortable while the body works to defeat the virus. Use whatever over-the-counter medications make the patient feel better, while not interfering with their ability to function. Local decongestants such as nasal sprays, systemic decongestants, and non-narcotic cough medications are very helpful. So is anti-inflammatory medication such as ibuprofen.

Equally important is maintaining fluid balance, eating well, staying warm, and getting enough rest. This reduces the number of stressors that the body has to deal with. The system will then be free to focus on fighting the virus and preventing a secondary bacterial invasion.

The patient with a persistent cough producing colored sputum usually needs antibiotics. If you are equipped with these drugs and know which ones to use, the patient can safely be treated in the field if they are otherwise okay. But the availability of antibiotics should not cause you to delay the evacuation of a patient with a serious problem. ✚

Chapter 30

Dental Problems

Teeth become a problem when they are fractured or knocked out. They become a nightmare when infected. Not only is there pain, but the pain can interfere with eating and drinking, which is essential to survival. Anyone planning an extended wilderness trip or ocean passage should have any potential problems checked by a dentist before departure.

With the trauma patient remember that loose teeth, or pieces of teeth, can result in airway obstruction. Damage to teeth can be associated with head and neck injury. Pain can produce acute stress reaction. Swallowing blood can cause vomiting.

The assessment of dental trauma is first directed at ensuring that potential critical body system problems are considered and stabilized. Beyond that, broken teeth do not represent a medical emergency.

Fractured Teeth

Anticipate:

- Infection
- Pain

Treatment:

- Pain medication
- Clean and cover with dental wax
- See dentist ASAP

Treatment of Dental Trauma: First, remove knocked-out or fractured teeth that might obstruct the airway. Position the patient to allow drainage of blood and debris from the mouth rather than down the throat. If the patient is awake and coopera- tive, have him rinse his mouth with cool water. This will clean out blood clots and loose teeth and help to stop bleeding. Examine the mouth with a flashlight. Look for teeth that are loose or fractured but still in the socket. Look for empty sockets that could match any knocked-out teeth you may have found.

Teeth that have been cleanly knocked out have a fair chance of reattaching if returned to their socket within an hour or so, the sooner the better. Try not to handle the tooth by its root; you will disturb the attachment fibers. Rinse the tooth in clean water and push it gently all the way back into its socket. You can splint the tooth to a healthy one with dental wax or temporary filling material. Any teeth that are very loose but still in the socket may be splinted in this manner as well.

Fractured teeth that are still in place are often extremely sensitive on exposure to air if the nerve is still alive. The open site can be treated with topical oral pain relievers such as oil of cloves and covered temporarily with dental wax or temporary filling material from a dental emergency kit.

The loss of a filling can be treated the same way using wax or filling material to protect the sensitive nerve tissue that is exposed when the filling falls out. If you don't have wax or filling material, loose fillings or crowns can be temporarily glued back in place with toothpaste. The patient should eat only soft foods and cool liquids.

Of course, any mouth held together with wax and toothpaste needs to see a dentist. This need not be on an emergency basis unless pain cannot be controlled. With broken or avulsed teeth, infection is an important anticipated problem. Antibiotics, usually penicillin, are often given to prevent it.

"Toothache" usually describes the pain experienced when an infection develops inside the tooth and at the base of the root. Bacteria enter through a break in the enamel caused by trauma or a cavity and form an abscess with the typical swelling, pressure, and pain. Swelling of the gum on the affected side may be evident, as well as tenderness of one or more teeth when tapped with a finger or stick. The infection may remain localized, or spread into the adjacent bone or sinus. In either case, it will be extremely uncomfortable. Both the infection and the pain it causes will be difficult to manage in the field.

Treatment of Dental Infection: The treatment of a dental infection includes drainage, antibiotics, and pain relief. Up until quite recently in dental history, drainage was invariably performed by pulling the tooth. The preferred method today is drilling and cleaning the inside of the tooth and installing a filling. Antibiotics are used to bring the infection under control, and pain relievers are usually necessary. What this means to you in the field is as simple as it is unfortunate: You need a dentist. Temporary pain relief may be obtained with oral topical pain relievers and aspirin or ibuprofen. If you carry antibiotics, a five-to-seven-day course may reduce the severity of the infection pending evacuation to dental care. ✚

Chapter 31

Eye Problems

The common terms "red eye," "pink eye," or "conjunctivitis" refer to inflammation of the thin, membranous lining of the eye and the inside of the eyelids (conjunctiva). There are a number of causes of conjunctival inflammation including infection, sunburn, sand in the eye, dirty contact lenses, trauma, chemical irritation, or even fatigue. It can also represent one of the symptoms of a more serious condition like glaucoma.

All the various causes of conjunctivitis produce similar symptoms. The patient will complain of an itching or burning sensation, tearing, and photophobia (discomfort caused by bright lights). The white of the eye will be covered with the enlarged blood vessels of the inflamed conjunctiva. In milder cases the cornea will remain clear. The pupil will continue to react to light. Vision will be unaffected except for transient blurring caused by tears or yellow exudate. Normal eye movements might be uncomfortable but fully intact.

Eye Problems

- *Conjunctival abrasion*
- *Corneal ulceration*
- *Corneal abrasion*
- *Glaucoma*
- *Foreign body*
- *Conjunctivitis*
- *Penetrating injury*
- *Etc.*

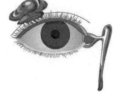

Serious or Not Serious?

In more severe cases there may be clouding of the cornea, persistent visual disturbances, and severe headache. Causes of conjunctivitis include:

Foreign Body—Sand or other debris that gets onto the conjunctiva will cause immediate irritation, redness, and tearing. Onset is usually abrupt, and the cause often obvious.

Corneal Abrasion—The clear center structure of the eye can be scratched by a foreign body, branch, fingernail, or windblown ice crystals. The cornea is structurally tough but exquisitely sensitive and will experience considerable pain and inflammation, making the patient feel like something is in the eye.

Sunburn—Ultraviolet light can burn the conjunctiva and cornea as it does unprotected skin. The result is the same: pain, redness, and sometimes swelling. Exam will reveal that the inflammation is limited to the sun-exposed part of the eye, leaving the conjunctiva under the lids unaffected. In severe cases the cornea may become pitted and cloudy in appearance in the condition known as snow blindness.

Infection—This is what most medical practitioners mean by the term "conjunctivitis." Bacteria invade the conjunctiva, causing the typical signs and symptoms of infection. The patient may notice yellow discharge that can stick the eyelids together during sleep. The eyelids themselves may appear slightly puffy and reddened. Vision will be blurred by tears and pus, but otherwise unaffected. Pain will be annoying but not severe. The cornea remains clear, pupils respond normally to light, and the eye moves without restriction.

Eye Problems

Red Flags:

- Vision impaired
- EOM impaired
- Unequal pupils
- Hyphema
- Severe eyelid swelling
- Penetrating foreign body
- Severe headache

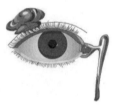

Chemical Irritation—Soap, dirty contact lenses, and stove fuel all cause chemical conjunctivitis. In mild cases the cornea remains clear. In severe cases it may be pitted or cloudy in appearance.

Treatment of Conjunctivitis: The generic treatment for conjunctival irritation includes pain medications, lubricating eyedrops, and protective lenses. Antibiotic eyedrops or ointment is applied when infection is present or anticipated. An eye patch is used only when eye movements will cause further harm, such as with an embedded or penetrating foreign body.

The easiest and most comfortable way to remove something like sand from the eye is by irrigation with water. The simplest method is to have the patient immerse his face in clean water and blink his eyes. Don't forget to have him hold his breath while doing this. You can also irrigate the eyes with your water bottle.

If the patient continues to have the sensation of something in the eye, you will need to do a more complete examination. Gently pull the lid away from the eye and use a bright light while the patient looks in all directions. If you find something, use a wet cotton swab or corner of a gauze pad to lift it off the membrane. If the object is embedded in the conjunctiva or cornea and resists your efforts to remove it, leave it alone. Embedded foreign bodies require medical attention. Patch the eye if safe to do so, and plan to walk out. Beware of using a patch in situations where impaired vision could be dangerous.

The cornea, which is the clear structure over the pupil, is structurally tough but neurologically sensitive. A corneal abrasion will often be visible with a flashlight shining across the eye from the side. Corneal abrasions are usually more annoying than serious. As long as no red flags are present, treatment may be generic and symptomatic with lubricating drops, pain medication, and protective lenses. Healing usually occurs within seventy-two hours. Sunburn is treated the same way.

Most mild bacterial and viral conjunctivitis will resolve spontaneously, but this is difficult to predict. You should allow the eyes to drain. Do not use a patch. Field treatment using frequent irrigation and warm soaks may improve the symptoms. Treatment with antibiotics is preferred. Severe infection evidenced by severe pain and eyelid swelling warrants an urgent evacuation.

Eye Problems

Generic Treatment:

- Sunglasses or goggles
- Irrigation and lubrication
- Antibiotic eye drops
- NSAIDs
- Pain free activity
- Red Flags = Evacuation

Note that pink eye can be quite contagious. Instruct your group to avoid sharing towels, goggles, or face masks. If you have access and authorization for antibiotic drops or ointment, treat both eyes.

The treatment for chemical exposure is copious irrigation with water or saline solution. Expect mild redness following prolonged irrigation, but it should begin to resolve within several hours following treatment. If it gets worse, the chemical may still be present. Irrigation should be repeated and evacuation considered.

Contact lenses are another frequent cause of inflammation, especially at altitude. Dry air and reduced oxygen tension can cause corneal damage. Affected patients should use lubricating eyedrops and allow their eyes as many lens-free hours per day as possible. In cases of infection or chemical exposure, contact lenses should be removed and discarded. ✚

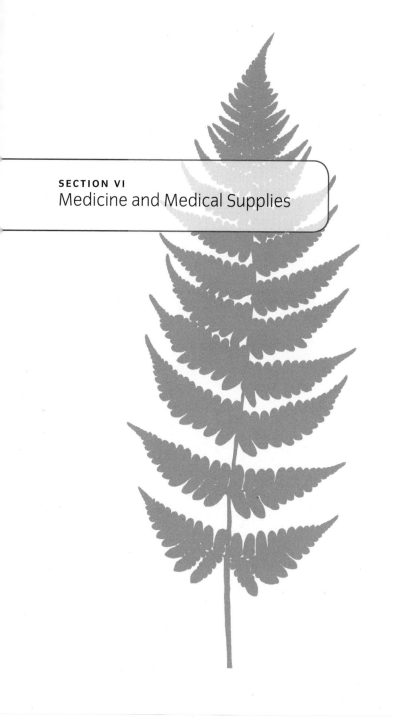

Chapter 32

Pain and Pain Medication

Pain is essential to survival. It provides guidelines for the safe and efficient use of our bodies and an early warning of serious trouble. It is the negative reinforcement that keeps us from doing bodily harm and serves to restrict mobility and prevent further damage after injury. It would be dangerous to eliminate pain completely.

The best treatment for pain is to treat the problem. Simple first-aid techniques will go a long way toward pain relief. The body rewards good treatment by hurting less. The use of drugs to control pain should be viewed only as an adjunct to the definitive treatment of the problem.

The Treatment of Pain

Treat the Cause:

- Reduce swelling.
- Realign fractures and dislocations.
- Adjust splints.

Treat the Symptoms:

- Ice.
- Analgesics (pain medication)
- Anesthetics ("numbing" agents)

Most analgesic (pain relieving) medications can be divided into three general groups: NSAIDs, other non-narcotic analgesics, and narcotics. Narcotics exert their analgesic effect on the central nervous system. They relieve pain by suppressing the brain's ability to perceive it. Pain impulses are still being sent along the nerve pathways from the site of injury, but the intensity is dulled at the receiving end. Examples of narcotics include morphine, codeine, and meperidine.

As a related effect, narcotics also depress mental function, respiration, and intestinal motility. When you're hurting, narcotics make you feel less pain, but they also make you stupid, clumsy, drowsy, and constipated. This may not be an issue

Narcotics

- Depress central nervous system
- May cause stomach upset and constipation
- Does not inhibit blood clotting
- Does not reduce swelling and inflammation
- Available in oral, transmucocal, sublingual, and injectable forms
- Eg: sublingual morphine, oral hydrocodone transmucosal fentanyl
- Require prescription and authorization

in the comfort and safety of your own home, but it can be a real problem halfway across the Pacific or high in the mountains somewhere. Narcotics are certainly useful, but the risks often outweigh the benefits.

A better choice for most acute pain situations are the NSAIDs (nonsteroidal anti-inflammatory drugs) because they don't cause central nervous system depression. NSAIDs exert their pain-relieving effect at the site of injury by reducing the stimulation of pain receptors in peripheral nerves and by reducing inflammation and swelling. The brain is wide awake and able to perceive pain, but there are

NSAIDs

- Work at the site of injury
- Do not depress central nervous system
- Reduces pain, fever, and inflammation
- Can cause stomach upset and inhibit clotting

Typical adult dose:

- ibuprofen: 400 – 800 mg q8h
- naproxen sodium: 250 – 500 mg q12h
- aspirin: 650 mg q4 – 6h

"The primary...side effect of NSAIDS is stomach irritation...take with food or antacids."

fewer pain impulses being sent. The granddaddy of all NSAIDs is aspirin, which is why they are also referred to as "aspirin-like drugs." Examples include ibuprofen (brand: Advil, Motrin, Nuprin) and naproxen sodium (Aleve).

Because NSAIDs are related to aspirin, they are not given much credit as strong pain relievers. People just don't believe that something as easily available as aspirin could be very effective. But aspirin is an excellent pain reliever. So are ibuprofen and naproxen sodium, which are often used in hospitals as the only post-surgery pain relievers necessary.

The primary undesirable side effect of NSAIDs is stomach irritation. The best way to avoid it is to always take NSAIDs with food or antacids. People with stomach problems should use these drugs with care, always taking the lowest effective dose. NSAIDs should be discontinued if persistent stomach pain develops.

The various NSAIDs available come in a broad spectrum of analgesic, anti-inflammatory, and antipyretic (anti-fever) properties. Ibuprofen does all three quite well and is a good choice for an expedition medical kit. It does a good job with minor to moderate pain at 200 to 400 mg every eight hours but can be used at up to 800 mg every six hours for severe pain. Ibuprofen is often used to reduce swelling in sprains and tendinitis, as well as to reduce fever in illness.

Acetaminophen (brand: Tylenol) is one of the other popular non-narcotic analgesics and is effective at relieving moderate pain and fever but is not useful for swelling and inflammation. It is still worth carrying because it tends to cause less stomach upset than the NSAIDs. Even people who can't take ibuprofen can usually tolerate acetaminophen.

Acetaminophen

- Does not depress central nervous system
- Reduces pain and fever
- Does not cause stomach upset
- Does not inhibit blood clotting
- Does not reduce swelling and inflammation

<u>Typical adult dose:</u>
650 - 1000 mg q4 - 6 hours (max 4000 mg in 24 hours)

Any pain medication should be used in the lowest effective dose for the shortest time necessary to minimize side effects. Always ask about allergies; people who are allergic to aspirin may react to any NSAID. Often, however, they will tell you that they can take Advil, Tylenol, or similar drugs without problems.

Finally, remember that medical information gets old quickly. New drugs, and new uses and contraindications for existing drugs, are being introduced all the time. As you stock your medical kit, supplement any published information by talking with a medical practitioner or pharmacist. ✚

Chapter 33
Antiseptics and Antibiotics

Antiseptics (also called disinfectants) are toxic chemicals that are designed to kill anything they come into contact with. Iodine and hydrogen peroxide are common examples. To control their effect, we adjust the concentration, site of application, and duration of contact. In low concentrations antiseptics will do a nice job of killing bacteria, viruses, and amoebas without harming you.

In most cases the safest approach is to use low concentrations for long duration. This is the idea behind disinfecting drinking water with only a few drops of iodine per liter, left to stand for thirty minutes. You can drink water purified in this manner for a long time with no ill effects.

For irrigating open wounds the best practice is to use large quantities of a very dilute solution of antiseptic, or just clean water. A concentrated solution of iodine or peroxide would sterilize the wound faster and more completely, but it would kill lots of your body's cells in the process. The chances of wound infection would actually increase with all of those dead cells lying around.

"Full strength" iodine solutions (Betadine, Povidone) are really only 2 to 10 percent, but this is enough to kill unprotected tissue. It should be used only to clean intact skin around a wound or before surgery. It should be washed off as soon as possible. Hydrogen peroxide is usually supplied as a 3 percent solution. It is less lethal than iodine but should not be used full strength in wounds either.

One of the best forms of antiseptic is iodine ointment (e.g., povidone iodine ointment). This is a low concentration solution that can be left on a wound for long-term protection. The ointment is also water soluble, and a small dab will purify a liter of water for drinking or wound irrigation. It can be a handy substance to have around.

Antibiotics are a more sophisticated and selective way to kill bacteria. Their mechanism of action targets the specific life functions of a specific type of bacterial cell. Penicillin, for example, interferes with the ability of certain types of bacteria to construct a new cell wall during reproduction. While most antibiotics have side effects, killing large numbers of body cells is usually not one of them.

Individual antibiotics have a typical "spectrum" of activity; that is, they act against some bacteria but not others. "Broad-spectrum" antibiotics act against a wide variety of bacteria and are more useful when you don't know exactly what you're dealing with. You can prepare to cover just about any type of infection on a remote expedition by carrying only two or three broad-spectrum antibiotics in your kit. Because bacteria rapidly develop resistance to antibiotics, a particular drug's effectiveness changes monthly. New drugs are constantly being introduced. Ask an experienced medical practitioner for current recommendations.

One of the easiest ways to use antibiotics is in the form of antibiotic ointment (e.g., Bacitracin), available without prescription. It is used to treat or prevent superficial skin infections without damaging healing skin cells. Unlike iodine ointment, it cannot purify water. A prescription ointment called mupirocin (brand: Bactroban) has been shown to be as effective as oral antibiotics on some skin infections.

Unfortunately, while antibiotics are useful against cellular organisms such as bacteria and amoebas, they don't do a thing to your garden-variety virus. You can take penicillin until you're blue in the face and it won't help your cold a bit. There are currently very few drugs effective against viruses, and those available tend to be extremely expensive. But this too is changing. ✚

Chapter 34
Medical Kits

The marketing departments of most outdoor equipment suppliers count on the medical naivety of the general public and on our tendency to try to solve the problem with money. Dozens of types of kits are offered, most at prices vastly inflated over the value of their contents. You can do a lot better on your own.

By now, you know that the most important element of any first-aid kit is the knowledge and experience carried in your head. The equipment and supplies can be relatively simple and inexpensive. How much first-aid equipment you carry is a function of how you carry it, how many people you're responsible for, where you're going, and what you know.

There is no point in carrying anything you don't know how to use. If you're carrying it on your back, there is no reason to carry anything that can be improvised from something else. As a result, a first-aid kit for backpacking can be about the size of this book. Larger groups, or people traveling by vehicle, boat, or horse, have the luxury of carrying more complete supplies.

On most trips it makes sense to arrange your kit in modules. Put the materials used for minor maintenance and repair, like Band-Aids and moleskin, in a separate container. This module will have as much to do with preventing medical problems as treating them and should be easily accessible. It may work best for each person in a group to have their own. Because this part of the kit will get a lot of use and be the most exposed to damage from snow and rain, it should contain only a small supply. It can be replenished from the main expedition kit as needed.

Medications, like antibiotics and pain relievers, should be in another module. The best container is a crushproof, waterproof, plastic box. In large groups it should be carried by the trip leader or medical officer. It should contain instructions and precautions for the use of the drugs carried, as well as a small notebook for recording times and dosages. Any prescription medications should be accompanied by documentation from the prescribing practitioner, especially if you will be crossing international borders.

The largest module is the main expedition kit. Because it serves mostly as a supply dump for the smaller modules, its size depends on the length of the trip. It should also include infrequently used and specialized first-aid supplies and equipment. The type of container you put it in will be determined by how you travel. The ubiquitous 5-gallon joint compound bucket has performed beautifully as a waterproof container on Outward Bound pulling boats. A compressible dry bag is good for pack or hiking trips. In wet conditions it's a good idea to further protect supplies inside the main kit by dividing them up among several plastic bags.

Your local pharmacist can be a great resource in acquiring supplies. He can also help you repackage medications into vials much smaller than what the product comes in off the shelf. A pharmacist should also be willing to point out generic medications that are equal to the expensive brand-name stuff. Go in with your whole supply list, explain what you're doing, and ask for a bulk discount.

The following list is a recommended basic kit. You will need to modify it to suit the conditions you expect and your level of training, but resist the temptation to load up on a lot of unnecessary gear. Your expedition medical kit is not meant to stand alone; it is an integral part of your whole gear inventory and trip plan. You don't need to weigh your kit down with hot packs, cold packs, triangular bandages, air splints, flashlights, and signal mirrors. This is the stuff that makes the commercial kits so big and expensive. Most of the splints and slings can be improvised, and you are already carrying the "survival gear" somewhere else.

Expedition Medical Kit

Module One—Knowledge and Experience: Invest in at least a week of training in backcountry or marine medicine.

Module Two—Reference: Written material, like this book and others, that you like and understand. You can tear out and carry only the important pages.

Module Three—Minor Maintenance and Repair Kit:
- Sterile scalpel blade
- 2 4 x 4" sterile gauze dressings
- 2 2 x 2" sterile gauze dressings
- 1 2 x 2" gel dressing or moleskin for blisters
- 6 Band-Aids (gauze in clear membrane type is best)
- 1 roll 1" flexible adhesive tape (conforms and moves with the body)
- 1 small bottle or ampule of tincture of benzoin (makes the skin sticky to hold tape in wet or cold weather)
- 1 small tube povidone iodine ointment (antiseptic for abrasions, burns, and blisters. A small dab dissolved in a quart of water purifies it for drinking or wound irrigation.)
- 1 small bottle liquid soap
- 1 pair splinter forceps (small tweezers)
- 4" x 5-yard roll of vet wrap (used to hold dressings in place over wounds, as compression bandage, or to fix splints in place)
- 2 pair latex or vinyl gloves
- sunblock
- insect repellent

Module Four—Medications:

Nonprescription
- Small bottle of acetaminophen (Tylenol)
- Small bottle of ibuprofen (Advil)
- Stool softener (e.g., Colace)
- Package of Pepto-Bismol tablets
- Package of antacid tablets
- Cough and cold preparations as desired
- Diphenhydramine capsules (Benadryl)
- Dramamine or other medication for motion sickness

Prescription (discuss with your medical practitioner)
- Antibiotic tablets
- Antibiotic eye ointment or drops
- Epinephrine kit for severe allergy (EpiPen, Benadryl, prednisone)
- Medication for severe pain
- Medication for vomiting and diarrhea
- Steroid cream
- Diamox (if going to altitude)
- Malaria prophylaxis if needed

Module Five—Main Expedition Kit:
- Resupply materials for Module Three kits
- Sam Splint™ (flexible aluminum covered with foam, can be cut and bent for a variety of uses. The only splint worth carrying on your back)
- 4 diaper pins
- More 4″ vet wrap (good for wound care and compression, as well as improvised splinting)
- Large dressings for big wounds (sanitary napkins work well)
- Xeroform gauze dressings (a foil-wrapped dressing impregnated with antiseptic that is especially useful in the long-term care of open wounds)
- Dental kit (oil of cloves, temporary filling material, dental wax, toothpaste, dental floss)
- 100 feet of 6mm low stretch rope (if not carried elsewhere)
- Roll of 15 yards of duct tape (for litters and splints, also fixes tents, boots, and boats)
- A handful of big plastic cable ties (for improvised litters and general repair)
- 1 pair trauma scissors (cuts almost anything, including Sam Splint)
- 1 fine hemostat (good for picking rocks and dirt from wounds or extracting hooks from humans or fish)

- Low reading clinical thermometer
- Burn sheet (100 percent cotton shirt fresh from the dryer, in a plastic bag)
- Notebook and pencil
- Butane lighter (warms duct tape to stick well in cold weather)

Day-Use Personal First-Aid Kit
(fits in a hunting coat pocket)
Materials:
- 1 roll 1" tape
- 2 4 x 4" gauze pads
- 1 large dressing (sanitary napkin works well)
- 1 3" elastic bandage
- 5 Band-Aids
- 1 3 x 3" blister pad, e.g., Spenco Adhesive Knit or moleskin
- 1 pair examination gloves
- 2 diaper pins
- 1 pair splinter forceps
- 1 emergency flashlight if not carried elsewhere
- 1 lighter or waterproof matches
- 1 knife if not carried elsewhere
- 1 small container of liquid soap
- 1 tube of povidone iodine ointment
- 1 container of total sunblock
- 1 5-yard roll of duct tape (usually wrapped around the container itself)
- 4 200mg ibuprofen tablets

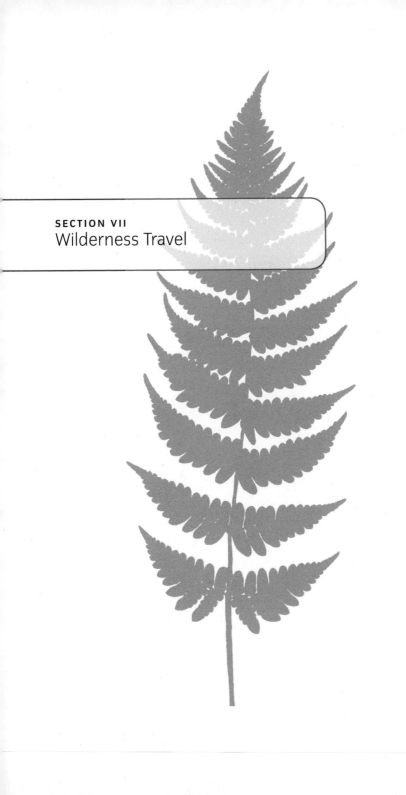

SECTION VII
Wilderness Travel

Chapter 35
Preparation for Wilderness Emergencies

The traditional view holds that the best preparation for medical emergencies is not to have them in the first place. I agree. There are plenty of how-to books on camping, sailing, canoeing, ice climbing, and so forth to help you do it right. Read them.

But because having medical emergencies is what *this* book is about, I'll take the statement a step further: The best time to have a medical emergency is when you're ready for it. Being ready means having the right attitude, knowledge, equipment, and margin of safety for the expedition or voyage you're planning.

Attitude, in my view, is the way one relates with the forces of the natural world. It is so much more peaceful to flow with natural trends than push against them. However, it is not always possible to go downriver, downhill, downwind, or with the tide. We tend to have schedules, destinations, and personal goals that put us in confrontation with nature.

Of course, challenging the elements can be great fun and an exhilarating experience. As long as you continue to feel that way, you'll be okay. However, one must beware of developing an adverse relationship with nature. This is a forewarning of serious trouble.

When it starts raining on *you*, or the wind shifts just to make *you* angry, or the snow starts just because *it* knows you're almost at the summit, your attitude has become dangerous. In an emergency situation, a bad attitude is big trouble. It contributes to irrational behavior, poor judgment, and despair. When you feel the "attitude," it's time to change your plans and reestablish harmony with your surroundings.

Knowing how to handle medical emergencies is a product of both information and experience. Only by combining the two can you gain real competence in the art of wilderness medicine. The information is readily available in this book and others like it. The experience is more difficult to come by. A reasonable substitute, at least as a beginning, can be found in the form of a quality hands-on course taught for the backcountry setting.

Knowing what to expect of the environment you are entering is important, too. You need to research expected weather and terrain conditions as well as the possible extremes. You should identify possible evacuation routes in case of trouble and establish some means of communication. You will want to know where shelters, ranger stations, roads, water, and so forth are located.

Equipment for wilderness emergency care is surprisingly simple. The real first-aid kit is your knowledge and experience. The bandages, ointments, moleskin, and other items in your pack are just tools for minor maintenance and repair.

The margin of safety in wilderness travel is the most important factor of all. An accident or illness that befalls a group that is dry, warm, and well fed is a problem but usually not a crisis. But if the group is wet, chilled, and low on supplies, the situation could be entirely different. Even a minor injury at that point can easily be fatal.

When you're in the mountains, out to sea, or on the river, you should frequently ask yourself, "What would I do if something went wrong?" It sounds a little paranoid, but this is a great exercise for the traveler new to the backcountry. If your answers are not coming up clear and reasonable, you are beyond your margin of safety. As you gain experience, your awareness of your own margin of safety becomes part of you. You feel comfortable within it and uneasy outside it. Pushing your own limits then becomes a matter of choice rather than accident. ✚

Chapter 36
Rescue and Evacuation

As I review my writing, I realize how many times treatment plans call for "evacuation to medical care" as if it were as easy as catching a bus. In reality it is everything but easy, especially when the injured person is no longer able to walk. A wilderness rescue can be a most dangerous and difficult operation.

Outside of state and national parks and a few municipalities, there is little in the way of organized professional response to backcountry emergencies. The responsibility for wilderness rescue is assumed by a variety of officials depending on where you are. This might include the Warden Service, Coast Guard, local fire departments, police, or ambulance crews. The official response usually relies heavily on volunteer rescue teams, the National Guard, ski patrols, and other organizations and individuals to do the actual work.

In many cases a rescue will be a well-coordinated effort by competent officials and well-trained volunteers. In others, the effort can be disorganized, inefficient, and downright dangerous. Either can happen depending on where you are, the situation you're in, and even the day of the week.

In spite of this inconsistency, it is not a situation that merits much complaint. As backcountry travelers and offshore sailors, we represent a minuscule portion of the general population. It is difficult to justify maintaining a sophisticated and expensive wilderness rescue system for so few people.

To enter the wilderness is to accept a much greater degree of personal responsibility. We must be able to get ourselves out of trouble whenever possible. Lacking that, we must be able to be of the greatest possible assistance to those who are coming to help us.

When you have stabilized a medical problem as best you can and have decided that outside help will be required, your communication skills become critical. Presenting a clear picture of the situation will allow rescuers to best apply their own local knowledge, experience, and resources to helping *you* solve *your* problem. This is where your SOAP note really becomes valuable. Not only has it helped you organize your thoughts but it can now provide the basis for organizing an evacuation. This is true whether you communicate by radio, telephone, carrier pigeon, or by sending a runner with a note.

Your SOAP note should include information about the scene. Describe the general condition of the group, weather and terrain conditions, and the status of food supplies and shelter. Try to stick to facts as much as possible. Avoid value judgments such as, "Oh my God, it's really bad, come quick!" This provides no useful information and only distracts people from a good planning process.

Recognize that any good rescue team is trained to perform their own survey of the scene and the patient's condition. Their assessment may differ from yours. Work with them, pointing out elements of your assessment that will help form a reasonable plan. This is no time for arguing. In all but the most unusual cases, when you've asked for rescue, the rescuers are in charge.

Responding to a medical emergency can be done by bringing the medical resources to the patient, or the patient to the medicine. Usually, it is a combination of the two. For example, rescue teams may bring intravenous fluids and oxygen to assist in stabilizing a patient during the carry-out. For the most part, though, the patient needs to return to civilization for definitive care.

The urgency with which this happens is a function of the patient's condition and the resources and skills available. It also hinges on your ability to distinguish real emergencies from logistical dilemmas. Very few backcountry situations really justify an all-out rapid evacuation. Only those injuries that involve a major problem with a critical body system deserve a major evacuation. Anything else can be more controlled, less desperate, and a lot less trouble. ✚

Appendix

Water Treatment

The term "disinfect" means to kill or remove living organisms such as bacteria, protozoa, algae, and viruses. To "purify" implies removing all foreign material including chemicals and minerals as well as life: a much more difficult process. In the wilderness setting where surface water is not subject to industrial contamination, our goal is usually just to eliminate disease-causing microorganisms.

Boil: Just bringing water to a boil disinfects it enough for drinking.

Chemicals: Double the time if the water is cold. Double the dose if the water is cloudy.

   a. **Iodine Tincture (2 percent):** Use two to five drops of tincture per liter of water and let stand for thirty minutes.
   b. **Iodine Tablets:** One tablet per quart of water and let stand for thirty minutes.
   c. **Chlorine:** Two drops of pure laundry bleach per quart of water; let stand for thirty minutes.

Filters: To prevent clogging, pre-filter the water through a cloth to remove large sediment. Note: The typical 0.2 micron filter does not remove viruses (e.g., hepatitis). If the filter you are using does not include a virucidal agent like an iodine cartridge, treat any water subject to fecal contamination with iodine or chlorine. Activated charcoal filters are capable of removing some chemical pollutants and sediment not affected by boiling. They will also remove the taste of chlorine or iodine after disinfection.

UV Radiation: Exposes the water to ultraviolet light for a prescribed period of time (e.g., Sterilight).

Glossary

Abbreviations, Acronyms, and Mnemonics

A: Problem list
A': Anticipated problem
A and O: Awake and oriented
APAP: Acetaminophen
AVPU: Awake
Verbal stimulus response
Painful stimulus response
Unresponsive
ALS: Advanced life support
ASA: Aspirin
BLS: Basic life support
BSA: Body surface area
CC: Chief complaint
C/MS: Level of consciousness and mental status
CNS: Central nervous system
c/o: Complains of
CPR: Cardiopulmonary resuscitation
CSM: Circulation, sensation, and movement
CVA: Cerebro-vascular accident (stroke)
EMS: Emergency medical services
HACE: High-altitude cerebral edema
HAPE: High-altitude pulmonary edema
Hx: History
ICP: Intracranial pressure
IM: Intramuscular
IV: Intravenous
mg: Milligram; 1/1000 of a gram
MI: Myocardial infarction (heart attack)
MOI: Mechanism of injury
NSAIDs: Nonsteroidal anti-inflammatory drugs
O: Objective
O₂: Oxygen
P: Plan
PAS: Patient assessment system
PFA: Pain-free activity
RF: Red flag

RICE:	Rest
	Ice
	Compression
	Elevation
Rx:	Treatment or prescription
S:	Subjective
SAMPLE:	Symptoms
	Allergies
	Medicines
	Past history of medical problems
	Last meal
	Events leading up to injury
SC:	Subcutaneous; under the skin
SOB:	Shortness of breath
SOAP:	Subjective—Information gained by questioning
	Objective—Information gathered during examination of the patient
	Assessment—List of problems discovered
	Plan—What is to be done about each problem
SX:	Symptoms
S/SX:	Signs and symptoms
TBI:	Traumatic brain injury
TIP:	Traction into position
VS:	Vital signs (with time recorded)
	BP: Blood pressure
	R: Respiratory rate
	T: Core temperature
	C: Level of consciousness (mental status if awake)
	S: Skin
	P: Pulse

General Glossary

Abrasion: Superficial wound that damages only the outermost layers of skin or cornea.

Abscess: A localized infection isolated from the rest of the body by inflammation.

Acute stress reaction (ASR): Autonomic nervous system controlled response to stress that can cause severe but temporary and reversible changes in vital signs.

Airway: The passage for air exchange between the alveoli of the lungs and the outside. Most commonly refers to the upper airway, including the nose, mouth, and trachea.

Altitude illness: The constellation of symptoms produced by altitude adjustment, high-altitude cerebral edema, and high-altitude pulmonary edema. Can be mild, moderate, or severe.

Alveoli: Membranous air sacks in the lungs where gas is exchanged with the blood.

Amnesia: Loss of memory.

Anaphylaxis: Systemic allergic reaction involving generalized edema of all body surfaces, vascular shock, and respiratory distress.

Angina: The pain of myocardial ischemia. Also called Angina pectoris. May be stable or unstable.

Antibiotic: A drug that selectively kills or interferes with the function or reproduction of bacteria.

Anticipated problems (A'): Problems that may develop over time as a result of injury, illness, or the environment.

Antifungal: A drug that selectively kills or interferes with the function or reproduction of pathogenic fungus.

Antiviral: A drug that selectively kills or interferes with the function or reproduction of viruses.

Arrhythmia: Abnormal heart rhythm. Also called a dysrhythmia.

Aspiration: Inhaling foreign liquid or other material into the lungs.

Basic life support (BLS): The generic process of supporting the functions of the circulatory, respiratory, and nervous systems using CPR, bleeding control, and spine stabilization.

Blood pressure cuff: Also known as a sphygmomanometer. Used for measuring blood pressure.

Capillaries: The smallest blood vessels in body tissues where gases and nutrients are exchanged between tissue cells and the circulating blood.

Cardiac arrest: Loss of effective heart activity.

Cardiogenic shock: Shock due to inadequate pumping action of the heart.

Cardiopulmonary resuscitation (CPR): A technique for artificially circulating oxygenated blood in the absence of effective heart activity. Includes positive pressure ventilation (PPV) and chest compressions.

Carotid pulse: The pulse felt on the side of the neck at the site of the carotid artery.

Cartilage: Connective tissue on the ends of bones at joints that provide a smooth gliding surface.

Central nervous system: The brain and spinal cord.

Cervical spine: The section of the spine in the neck between the base of the skull and the top of the thorax.

Cold challenge: The combined cooling influence of wind, humidity, and ambient temperature.

Cold response: The normal body response to the cold challenge, including shell/core effect and shivering.

Compartment syndrome: Swelling within a confined body compartment, like the connective tissue compartments in the leg or inside the skull. Can cause loss of local perfusion (ischemia) resulting in death of tissue (necrosis).

Compensation: Involuntary changes in body functions designed to maintain perfusion pressure and oxygenation of vital body tissues in the presence of injury or illness.

Concussion: Brain injury. May be mild or severe. Also called head injury or traumatic brain injury.

Conjunctiva: The membrane covering the white of the eye and the inner surfaces of the eyelids.

Conjunctivitis: Inflammation of the conjunctiva due to irritation, infection, or injury. Most often used in reference to infection (pink eye).

Cornea: The clear part of the eye over the iris and pupil.

Cornice: An overhanging drift of snow formed as wind blows over a ridge or mountaintop.

Crepitis: The feel or sound of bones or cartilage grating when moved. Typical at the site of an unstable fracture. Can also describe the feel or sound of subcutaneous air when palpated.

Cyanosis: The blue color seen in the lips and skin of a patient with poor tissue oxygenation. This is actually the color of deoxygenated hemoglobin.

Debridement: Wound cleaning, including removal of foreign material and devitalized tissue.

Definitive treatment: Therapy that cures the disease or corrects the problem.

Dental abscess: Infection at the base of a tooth.

Diagnosis: The identification of a medical problem by name. May be generic or specific.

Diaphragm: Muscle at the lower end of the chest cavity that contracts to create a vacuum, which draws air into the lungs. The diaphragm works with muscles of the chest wall, shoulders, and neck to perform ventilation.

Discharge: Fluid escaping from the site of infection or inflammation. Also called exudate.

Dislocation: Disruption of normal joint anatomy.

Distal: An anatomical direction; away from the body center. The wrist is distal to the elbow.

Dysrhythmia: An abnormal heart rhythm. Also called arrhythmia.

Edema: Swelling due to leaking of serum from capillaries.

Epinephrine: The synthetic form of the hormone adrenalin. Used to constrict blood vessels and dilate airway tubes.

Evacuation: Transferring a patient from the scene of injury or illness to definitive medical care.

Extension: Movement at a joint that extends an extremity away from the center of the body. The opposite of flexion.

Extrication: Removing or freeing a patient from entrapment or confinement.

Exudate: Discharge.

Femoral artery: Large artery that travels along the femur in the thigh.

Femur: Long bone of the thigh.

Flail chest: The loss of rigidity of the chest wall due to multiple rib fractures.

Flexion: Movement of a joint that brings the extremity closer to the body. The opposite of extension.

Focused history and physical exam: The third stage in the patient assessment system, which includes the examination of the whole body, SAMPLE history, and vital signs.

Fracture: Broken bone, cartilage, or solid organ.

Frostbite: Frozen tissue. May be partial thickness or deep.

Frostnip: Loss of circulation due to the vasoconstriction of blood vessels in the skin during the early stages of tissue freezing. Also called superficial frostbite.

Glaucoma: Disease or condition causing increased pressure within the globe of the eye.

Head injury: Injury to the brain. Also called concussion.

Heart attack: Heart muscle ischemia caused by a blood clot or spasm of the coronary arteries, or an arrhythmia, resulting in the necrosis (or infarction) of heart tissue.

Heat challenge: Combined effects of ambient temperature and metabolic activity, which contribute to body heating.

Heat exhaustion: Compensated volume shock caused by fluid loss due to sweating.

Heat response: The normal body response to the heat challenge, including sweating and vasodilation of the shell.

Heat stroke: Severe elevation of body temperature (above 40 degrees C).

Hemothorax: Blood in the chest cavity as a result of injury, usually collecting between the chest wall and lung tissue.

Hyperextension: To extend a joint beyond its normal range of motion.

Hyperventilation syndrome: Respiratory alkalosis. The nervous system symptoms of numbness, visual field contraction, and light-headedness caused by reduced carbon dioxide in the blood due to excessive ventilation, usually associated with acute stress reaction.

Hypoglycemia: Low blood sugar.

Hypothermia: Below normal body core temperature (37 degrees C).

Infarction: Tissue death due to loss of perfusion and oxygenation. Necrosis.

Infection: Pathologic colonization of body tissues by bacteria, virus, fungus, or other micro-organisms.

Inflammation: A generic body response to illness or injury resulting in redness, swelling, warmth, and tenderness.

Initial assessment: The second stage of the patient assessment system, and the initial examination of the patient. Looks for life-threatening problems with the critical functions of the circulatory, respiratory, and nervous systems.

Intoxication: Altered level of consciousness or mental status due to the influence of chemicals such as drugs, alcohol, and inhaled gases.

Intracranial: Inside the skull (cranium).

Intravenous fluids: Fluids infused directly into the circulatory system through a hypodermic needle inserted into a vein, usually used to temporarily increase the volume of circulating blood or restore fluid lost to sweating or diarrhea.

Intubation: Placing an endotrachial tube into the trachea.

Involuntary guarding: Refers to abdominal muscle spasm to protect the abdomen from painful movement. Considered a sign of peritoneal irritation.

Ischemia: Lack of local perfusion to body tissues. Can be caused by a clot, constriction, shell core effect, or tight splint. Persistent ischemia will result in infarction.

Level of consciousness: Describes the level of brain function in terms of responsiveness to specific stimuli (the AVPU Scale): A = Awake, V = responds to Verbal stimuli, P = responds to Painful stimuli, U = Unresponsive to any stimuli.

Ligaments: Tough connective tissue joining bone to bone across joints.

Local effects: Effects that are restricted to the immediate area of injury or infection (versus systemic effects).

Long bones: Bones that have a long structural axis such as leg and arm bones as opposed to flat bones like ribs and shoulder blade.

Lower airway: Trachea, bronchi, alveoli.

Lumbar spine: The lower section of the spine between the thorax and the pelvis.

Mechanism of injury (MOI): The cause of injury, or a description of the forces involved.

Mental status: Describes the level of brain function in an awake patient (A on AVPU) in terms of memory, orientation, level of anxiety, and behavior.

Mid-range position: Position in a joint's range of motion between full extension and full flexion. Also called neutral position.

Near drowning: At least temporary survival of water inhalation.

Neutral position: The position approximately halfway between flexion and extension. Also called the mid-range position.

Open fracture: Fracture with an associated break in the skin. Also called a compound fracture.

Oxygenation: To saturate blood with oxygen in the lungs. Also describes the transfer of oxygen from the blood to body cells (cellular oxygenation).

Parasthesia: Neurological deficit, usually described as weakness or numbness and tingling.

Patella: Kneecap.

Pathologic: Harmful to the body. Usually used to describe bacteria, fungus, or virus.

Patient assessment system: A system of surveys including Scene Size-Up, Primary Survey, and Secondary Survey designed to gather information about an injured or ill patient and the environment in which he or she is found.

Perfusion: The passage of blood through capillary beds in body tissues.

Peripheral nerves: The nerves running between body tissues and the spinal cord.

Photophobia: Eye pain or headache caused by bright lights.

Pneumonia: Infection of lung tissue resulting in the accumulation of fluid in the alveoli.

Pneumothorax: Free air in the chest cavity, usually from a punctured lung or chest wall.

Polypro: Slang for polypropylene clothing.

Proximal: Toward the center of the body. The elbow is proximal to the wrist.

Pulmonary edema: Swelling of lung tissue resulting in the collection of fluid in the alveoli.

Rales: The noise produced by pulmonary edema. Sounds like crinkling cellophane or air being sucked through a wet sponge.

Reduction: Restoring a dislocated joint to normal position. Also restoring a displaced fracture to normal anatomic position.

Rhonchi: Sound produced by mucus or fluid in the lower airways.

Scene size-up: The first stage of the Patient Assessment System during which you look for dangers to the rescuer and patient, numbers of people injured, and the mechanism of injury.

Seizure: Uncoordinated electrical activity in the brain.

Sepsis: Systemic infection.

Serum: The liquid portion of the blood, as distinguished from blood cells and platelets.

Sexually transmitted disease (STD): Infection transmitted from person to person by sexual activity.

Shell/core compensation: Vasoconstriction in the skin and gut to shunt blood to vital body organs. Occurs as a result of volume shock and cold response.

Shell/core effect: A compensation mechanism seen in shock and cold response that reduces blood flow to the body shell in order to preserve perfusion and warmth in the vital organs of the core. Can also be reversed in core/shell effect.

Shock: Inadequate perfusion pressure in the circulatory system resulting in inadequate cellular oxygenation.

Signs: Response elicited by examination, e.g., pain when the examiner touches an injured area (tenderness).

Sinus: Hollow spaces in the bones of the skull.

Sinusitis: Inflammation of the membranous lining of the sinuses due to infection, allergy, or toxic exposure. Usually used in reference to infection.

Spasm: Involuntary contraction of muscle.

Spinal cord: The cordlike extension of the central nervous system encased within the bones of the spinal column, running from the base of the brain to the mid lumbar spine.

Spine: The column of bony vertebrae extending from the base of the skull to the pelvis. Includes the bones, ligaments, cartilage, and spinal cord.

Stethoscope: An instrument used to transmit body sounds directly to the ears of the examiner via rubber tubes.

Sublingual: Under the tongue. Usually refers to a route of medication administration such as a sublingual tablet of nitroglycerine or morphine.

Survey: A systematic examination of the scene and the patient.

Swelling: Abnormal fluid accumulation in body tissues due to bleeding or edema.

Symptomatic treatment: Therapy that relieves symptoms but does not necessarily treat the cause.

Symptoms: Condition described by the patient, e.g., pain on swallowing.

Synovial fluid: Joint fluid, lubrication inside a joint.

Systemic: Involving the entire body, such as a systemic infection or systemic allergy.

Tetanus: Nervous system spasm and paralysis caused by the toxin released by *Clostridium tetani* bacteria. Also called lockjaw.

Thorax: The chest, or chest cavity.

Tourniquet: A constricting band used to prevent or restrict the flow of blood to an extremity.

Toxin: Chemical that has a damaging effect on body tissues or the function of the nervous system.

Toxin load: The combined systemic effect of numerous small toxic exposures such as a large number of insect bites or man-of-war stings.

Traction: Tension applied along the long axis of an extremity.

Traction splint: A splinting device designed to maintain traction on an extremity, primarily used for femur fractures in the field setting.

Trauma: Injury.

Traumatic brain injury: Injury to the brain. Also called head injury or concussion.

Trench foot: Inflammation due to ischemia caused by cold-induced vasoconstriction during prolonged exposure to cold and wet conditions.

Umbilicus: Navel, belly button.

Universal precautions: Set of precautions or procedures to minimize the risk of disease transmission via contact with infected body fluids. Includes gloves, eye protection, face shields or masks, protective clothing, and the use of disinfectants. Universal precautions also includes proper procedures for handling and disposing contaminated articles and instruments.

Upper airway: Mouth, nose, throat (larynx).

Vapor barrier: A vapor-proof wrap or covering that prevents evaporative cooling.

Vascular bundle: A grouped nerve, artery, and vein following the same pathway.

Vascular shock: Shock due to dilation of blood vessels.

Vasodilation: Dilation of blood vessels.

Ventilation: The movement of air in and out of the lungs.

Vertebrae: The bones of the spine.

Vital signs: Measurements of body function including blood pressure, pulse, respiration, level of consciousness, skin color, and body core temperature.

About Outward Bound

Outward Bound, America's preeminent experiential education organization, was a pioneer in the field of wilderness experiential learning when it was established in the United States in 1961, and has continued to deliver unparalleled outdoor educational programs ever since. Today, Outward Bound provides adventure and learning in the wilderness, urban environments, the workplace, and schools, helping participants achieve their full potential and inspiring them to serve others and to care for the world around them.

A Brief History

Outward Bound is based on the educational ideas of Kurt Hahn, an influential German-born educator. Hahn established the School at Schloss Salem in an attempt to combat what he perceived as the deterioration of values in post-World War I Germany. Salem's progressive curriculum focused on character development through physical fitness, skill attainment, self-discipline, and compassionate service. In 1933, thirteen years after establishing Salem, Hahn fled Nazi-ruled Germany to Britain. Soon after his arrival, he set about establishing the Gordonstoun School in Scotland to continue his work under the motto, "Plus est en vous" ("You have more in you than you think").

In 1941, in a joint effort with British shipping magnate Sir Lawrence Holt, Hahn founded the first Outward Bound Sea School at Aberdovey, Wales. The school not only taught sailing skills, but also integrated Hahn's core belief that character development was just as important as academic achievement. Hahn's goal was to teach self-reliance, fitness, craftsmanship, and compassion as a way to prepare the youth of Great Britain to serve their nation in the struggle against Nazi Germany. The program revolved around a series of increasingly rugged challenges designed to develop the self-confidence, fortitude, and leadership skills required to survive harsh physical and mental challenges. The name of the school was adopted from the nautical term used when ships leave the safety of the harbor for the open sea: They were said to be "outward bound," bound for unknown challenges and adventures.

Josh Miner, an American who taught under Hahn at Gordonstoun, was inspired to bring Outward Bound to the United States. Working with a small group of committed supporters, Miner founded the Colorado Outward Bound School in 1961, bringing the principles of hands-on learning and compassionate service through outdoor adventure to America.

Outward Bound Today

Today Outward Bound has expanded to thirty-six countries throughout the world. In the United States, the organization serves over 25,000 participants in outdoor programs each year. Central to its mission is its scholarship program, designed to attract and benefit populations that are typically underserved. Within the public courses offered to individuals, approximately 25 percent of participants receive financial support, and 23 percent of all participants are ethnically diverse.

In the United States, to advance the goals of changing lives, building teams, and transforming schools, Outward Bound now offers the following programs and services:

- Traditional adventure-based wilderness courses
- Long-term teacher development and whole school reform
- Programs for at-risk youth and their families
- Urban area–based programs for students, educators, and civic leaders to develop a better understanding of their capabilities and value to their community
- Innovative leadership development for business and professional organizations

While most of Outward Bound's programming has been unified under a single board and management team, three organizations—North Carolina Outward Bound, Thompson Island Outward Bound, and New York City Outward Bound—operate under charters granted by Outward Bound USA and work closely with the affiliation.

Although the programs vary broadly in target population, setting, and objective, they all contain the basic elements that Kurt Hahn espoused as central to the development of effective and compassionate citizens: adventure and challenge; inclusion and diversity; social and environmental responsibility; learning through experience; character development; and compassion and service. For participants in any of the varied programs, in any part of the world, these six core values provide the foundation for their Outward Bound experience.

The Wilderness Instructors

Outward Bound instructors are highly trained, qualified educators and outdoor skills specialists. Participant safety is a high priority—integral to every program. Instructors are required to carry first-aid certification at the wilderness first-responder level, and many are emergency medical technicians. They are also proficient in—and passionate about—the specific wilderness skills of the activity they teach, whether rock climbing, sailing, mountaineering, or white-water rafting. To help participants along their personal growth paths, instructors are trained in managing groups and individuals. A vital component of every course is the instructors' ability not only to shepherd participants through individual course challenges but also to help them work as contributing members of a team while simultaneously assuming leadership roles.

Outward Bound's Lasting Impact

The impact of each active learning expedition extends well beyond the course itself. For some, it's demonstrated in improved school performance; for others, in closer relationships with family and friends; and for many, transformation is reflected in a new commitment to service. When Outward Bound participants return home, they bring with them a new sense of responsibility, an enhanced appreciation of the environment, and a strong service ethic that they share with friends and family, integrating what they learned into the fabric of their communities. In one participant's words, "What I was lacking I have found; now I have the tools to keep growing and to work hard to accomplish my dreams, and to do anything I can to help others accomplish their dreams as well." ✚

Index

About the Author

Jeffrey Isaac is an experienced physician assistant with a particular interest in remote and extreme environments. In twenty-five years in medical practice, he has served as an ambulance medic, fire/rescue crewman, professional ski patroller, and emergency department practitioner. He is a senior instructor with Wilderness Medical Associates and a former Outward Bound instructor and course director. He is also a licensed captain and an experienced blue water sailor, having logged thousands of miles in the Atlantic and Pacific Oceans and the Caribbean Sea.

While teaching on Hurricane Island in 1982, Isaac met with Dr. Peter Goth about the challenge of designing appropriate medical training for the Outward Bound instructors working there. They found common ground in a practical and commonsense approach to medicine and a depth of experience well suited to their task. Their early efforts set the stage for Dr. Goth's founding of Wilderness Medical Associates, Inc. and the pair's co-authorship of the first edition of *The Outward Bound Wilderness First-Aid Handbook*.

Isaac now lives in Crested Butte, Colorado, where he practices emergency medicine with the Crested Butte Medical Center and serves as team leader and medical officer for Crested Butte Search and Rescue. In addition to this publication, he is co-author of *Wilderness and Rescue Medicine, a Practical Guide for the Basic and Advanced Practitioner,* used as a text for Wilderness Medical Associates courses worldwide. ✚